A BEGINNER'S GUIDE TO NATIVE AMERICAN HERBAL MEDICINE

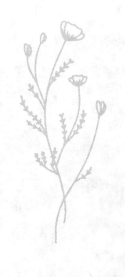

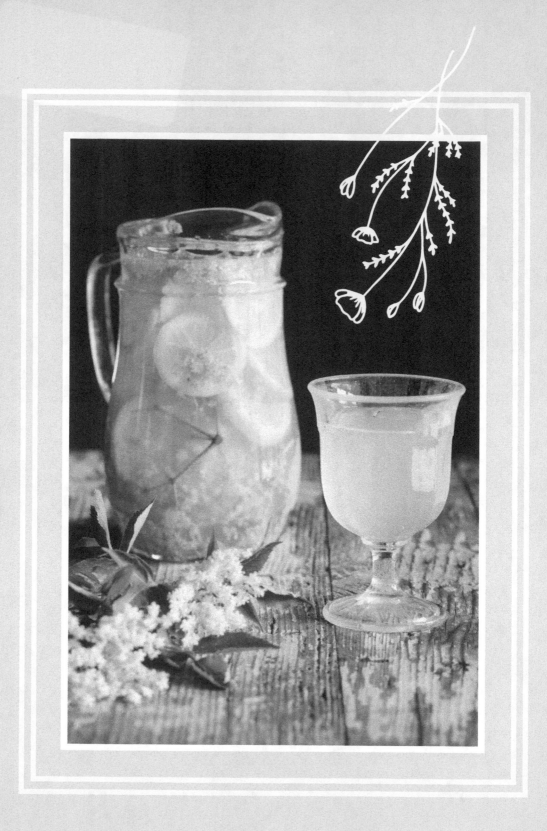

A BEGINNER'S GUIDE TO
NATIVE AMERICAN
Herbal Medicine

75 Natural Remedies
for Wellness and Balance

ANGELA LOCKLEAR QUEEN

ROCKRIDGE
PRESS

Copyright © 2023 by Rockridge Press

All rights reserved. No part of this publication may be reproduced, stored in a retrieval system, or transmitted in any form or by any means, electronic, mechanical, photocopying, recording, scanning, or otherwise, without the prior written permission of the Publisher. Requests to the Publisher for permission should be addressed to the Permissions Department, Rockridge Press, 1955 Broadway, Suite 400, Oakland, CA 94612.

First Rockridge Press trade paperback edition 2023

Rockridge Press and the Rockridge Press logo are trademarks or registered trademarks of Callisto Media Inc. and/or its affiliates in the United States and other countries and may not be used without written permission.

For general information on our other products and services, please contact our Customer Care Department within the United States at (866) 744-2665, or outside the United States at (510) 253-0500.

Paperback ISBN: 979-8-88650-127-8 | eBook ISBN: 979-8-88650-250-3

Manufactured in the United States of America

Interior and Cover Designer: Heather Krakora
Art Producer: Casey Hollister
Editor: Olivia Bartz
Production Editor: Ashley Polikoff
Production Manager: Lanore Coloprisco

Illustrations and photographs by:
Shutterstock: © Ludmila Ivashchenko: front cover left; © Chatham172: front cover right; © Merfin: (herb and floral illustrations); © mizy: v; © Merfin: throughout (cedar illustrations); © Nespola Designs: (wicker texture): 1; © Olga_Kop: 30; © Flower_Garden: 31; © damann: 32; © T-I: 33; © Corinne Prado: 34; © Sean Lema: 35; © alybaba: 36; © martin.dlugo: 37; © Ksenia Shestakova: 38; © Nick Pecker: 39; © Ksenz-E: 40; © KAISARMUDA: 41; © AnnaNel: 42; © Simon Groewe: 43, back cover; © Anastasiia Malinich: 44; © Real Moment: 45; © Robin T. Cowen: 46; © Dan4Earth: 47; © Nancy J. Ondra: 48; © Nadya So: 49; © imageBROKER.com: 50; © Cristina Ionescu: 51; © Sheila Fitzgerald: 52; © Julia Senkevich: 53; © Patrick Daxenbichler: 54; © shalom3: 55; © LifeisticAC: 56; © phichak: 57; © Sundry Photography: 58; © natalia bulatova: 60; © Jason Busa: 144
Stocksy: © Studio Serra: front cover second from left, ii; © Canan Czemmel: front cover second from right, x
© Hélène Dujardin: (wood background)
iStock/Getty Images: © Nataliia Sirobaba: 27, 59; © SusanSerna: 28

10 9 8 7 6 5 4 3 2

This book is dedicated to my family; without their sacrifice of my time and energy, I couldn't have been able to accomplish this goal.

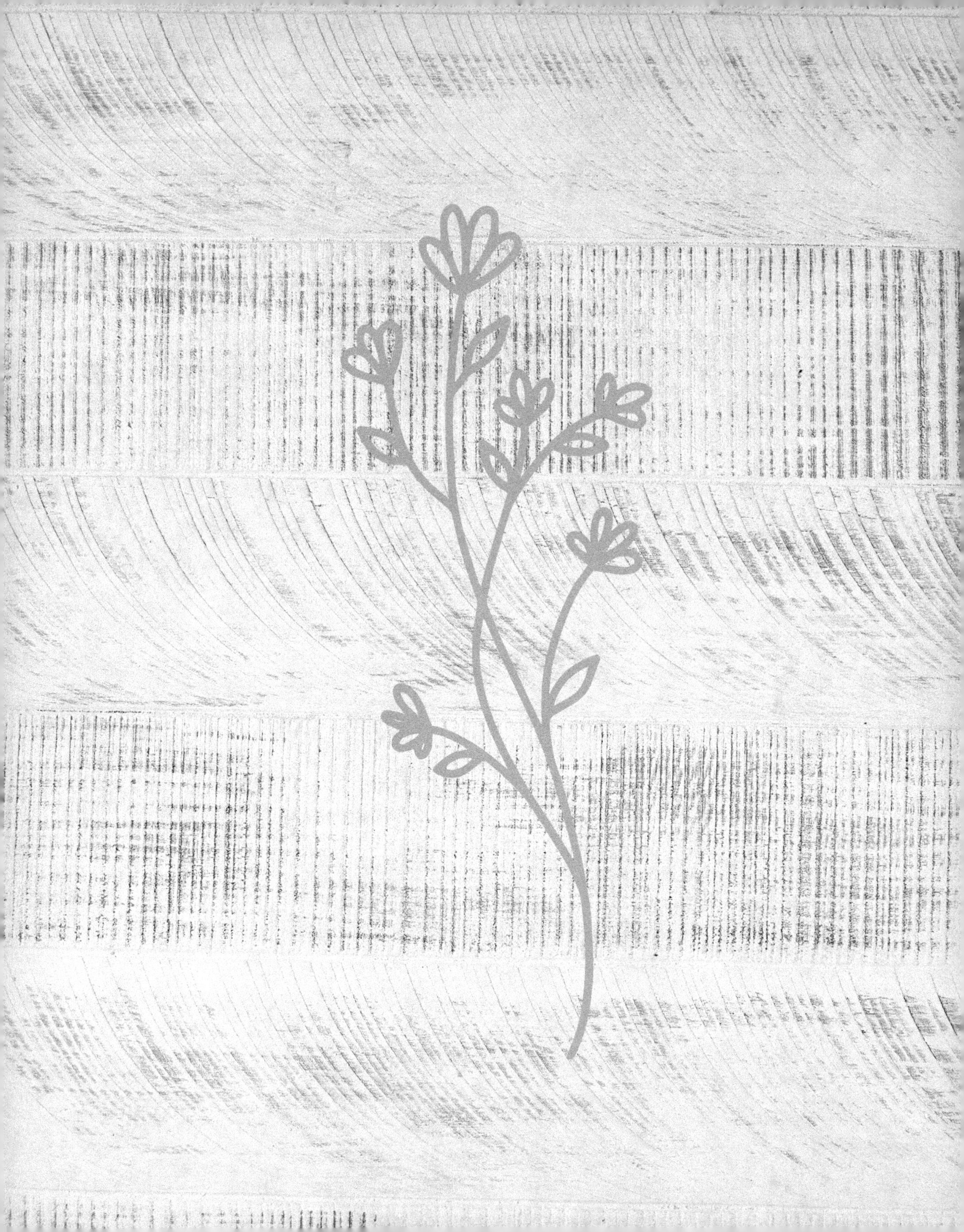

CONTENTS

Introduction viii

How to Use This Book ix

PART I:
Introduction to Native American Herbal Medicine   *1*

CHAPTER 1: *Understanding Native American Herbal Medicine* *3*

CHAPTER 2: *Preparing Your Tools and Ingredients* *17*

PART II:
Essential Herbs to Know   *29*

PART III:
Native American Remedies for Health and Wellness   *61*

Resources *145*

References *147*

Index *149*

INTRODUCTION

Choosing to be the writer of a book about Native American herbalism and sacred plants, even as an Indigenous person, calls for a pause. The complexities of being a BIPOC writer, especially in the spiritual and herbal spaces, carries weight. For me, honoring Native American communities is the highest priority. The opinions about sharing Native American traditional knowledge vary from one group to another. Many Indigenous peoples are protective of traditional knowledge due to historical trauma, whereas others believe we can heal the earth and ourselves by sharing the wisdom of our ancestors. I honor both sides, recognizing that Native American herbalists have been sharing their knowledge for decades, but in recent years, aspects of our culture have been significantly commodified, causing harm to Indigenous plants and traditions. With that said, as an Indigenous woman who has weaved herself in and out of herbalism spaces for almost twenty years, I have recognized there is a lack of Native American representation, and I hope to be part of shifting this imbalance for other Native American herbalists so they, too, can use their knowledge to make an income while protecting the parts of Indigenous culture that should be held in high regard.

Although many aspects of this book carry cultural richness, and other aspects are education offered by a trained herbalist, gardener, and wildcrafter, this book is also the knowledge of only one Native American woman from one tribe. I do not claim this space with the intention of representing all Indigenous peoples. My goal is to bridge the gap between culture and modern society so I can further educate on what harms cultural appropriation in wellness spaces can inflict on Native communities. Due to the commercialization of sacred Indigenous plants, it is not without discernment I chose to write about them. Because these plants capture so much interest, I believe they can channel important conversations about Indigenous culture. However, I don't condone the commercialized sale and promotion of the four sacred plants. Traditional ceremonies fall under the most sensitive of topics among Native Americans, so although I touch on them briefly through the lens of the four elements (earth, air, water, and fire), I personally regard them as too sacred to the tribes from which they come to write about them in detail. My belief is that non-Native people are drawn to traditional Indigenous practices because they perceive Indigenous peoples to be more deeply connected to the earth. However, we can all form a deeper relationship with the earth by understanding the four elements and how they show up in the world around us.

HOW TO USE THIS BOOK

This book is designed to allow you to toggle back and forth through the chapters, herb profiles, and herbal remedies. However, chapter 1 is fundamental to understanding herbalism through an Indigenous lens, because it touches on the history of Native American herbalism, how plants are currently used, and how understanding the elements (earth, air, water, and fire) can lessen cultural appropriation and offer healing through earth-based practices. Chapter 1 also includes herbal preparation methods that will be important once you gather your medicinal plants, making it a vital part of your introduction to herbalism.

If you're eager to learn how to procure the plants you'll need for these preparations, you might choose to look over chapter 2 first to learn more about wildcrafting, gardening, and buying herbs. Once you finish, pour yourself a cup of tea, and return to chapter 1. Either way, this book's information is fluid, and you can move through it depending on your specific needs or interests. The herb profiles are dense with information and may be visited when you want to learn about the history and uses of a specific plant. You may also find it necessary to bounce around the remedies based on the season and your physical needs, because they are arranged by ailment and in alphabetical order. Additionally, I've included many nutritious remedies that can become part of your everyday life for increased wellness, so be sure to look through them one by one, bookmarking those that excite you.

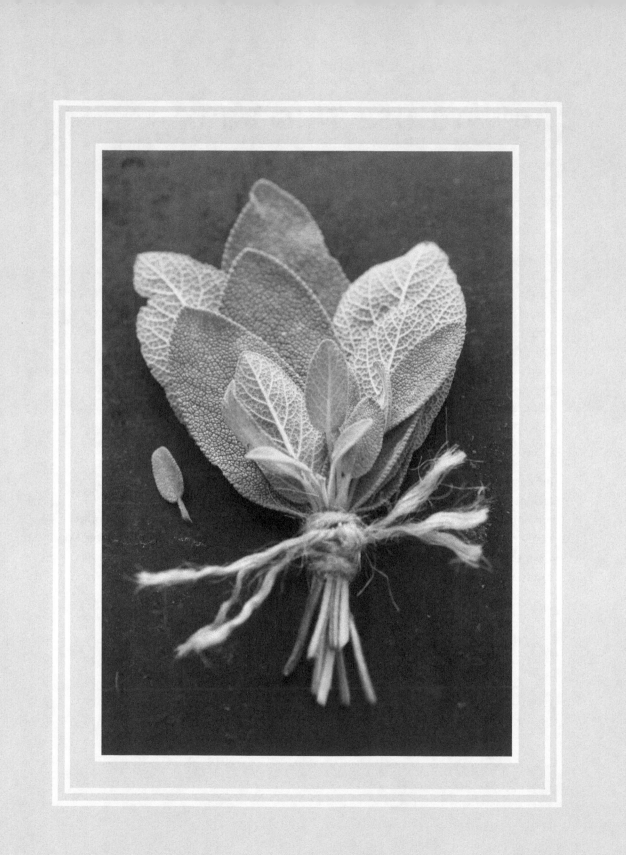

PART I

Introduction to Native American Herbal Medicine

Native Americans have been known to value medicinal plants more than gold itself and continue to value these plants as an inseparable part of their existence. Native American wisdom recognizes our reliance on the natural world to maintain optimum health and ward off even the worst of illness. Historically, Native Americans had knowledge of nearly every plant that grew around them, sharing this knowledge throughout tribes and benefiting physically, emotionally, and spiritually from these medicinal and nutritional plants. In chapters 1 and 2, you'll learn more about the relationship between Native Americans and these medicines of the earth and what they had to endure throughout history to retain their earth-based healing practices. The value of herbal medicine is a universal one that you can gain from when you learn the proper methods of using herbs in your day-to-day life. In these chapters, you'll acquire the knowledge to get you started. You'll also learn to forage plant medicines in a way that is reflective of how the First Peoples have always gathered plants. Native Americans also lived in agrarian societies, cultivating plants for the community. We discuss how growing your own herb garden is also a valid way to acquire your medicinal plants. This part ends with teaching you how to dry and store the herbs you have harvested.

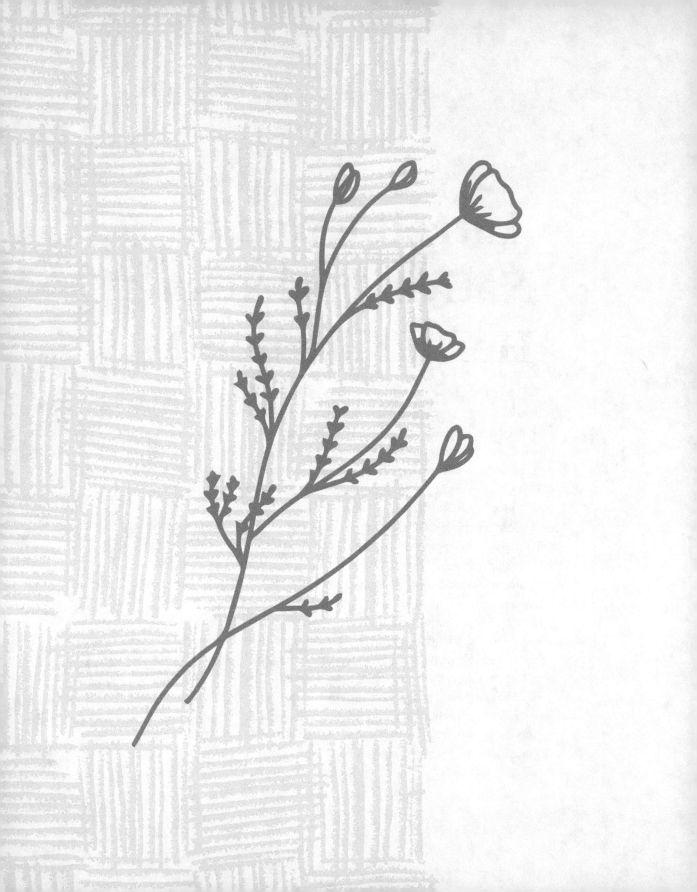

CHAPTER 1

Understanding Native American Herbal Medicine

This chapter offers an overview of how Native Americans learned to use regional plants for medicinal purposes by bearing witness to the natural world around them. We explore the Native American way of healing the whole body to reach grounded health, which considers the physical as well as the emotional and spiritual. In this chapter, you will also learn about sacred medicinal plants used during healing ceremonies. These plants are elevated above the rest and are often featured in many beautiful creation myths from various Native American tribes. Because of this deep reverence, it is impossible to write about these plants with the fullness they deserve.

This first chapter teaches the simplest of ways you can start incorporating plant medicine into your everyday life with little more than an herb and hot water. Traditions with such a long history can sometimes feel overwhelming. However, I hope that you simply feel encouraged to see the world around you in a new way that acknowledges your interconnectedness with all aspects of nature—including the rhythms of the seasons, the plants, the animals, and even the smallest of pebbles that shows up by your toe on a barefoot day.

The Origins of Native American Herbal Medicine

Herbalism describes the interactive relationship between medicinal plants and humans. For Native Americans, this relationship is one into which they are born. We know this from Indigenous creation myths about plants coming to life alongside Indigenous peoples. It is seen through the very foundation of how Native Americans have traditionally approached well-being. The health of the physical body is only one spoke on the wheel in Native American culture; health, for Native Americans, also encompasses the emotional, spiritual, and intellectual bodies.

It is believed that Native Americans came to know how plants could heal them and what plants were safe by observing the animals' instinct to consume plants when they fell ill. Before colonization, it is estimated that upward of one hundred million Native Americans in more than six hundred tribes were thriving on the North and South American continents. During those times, the vast amount of herbal knowledge was passed on through oral teachings and storytelling, but it was not officially documented. In John Lawson's book *History of North Carolina*, he wrote, "Among all the discoveries of America by the French and Spaniards; I wonder why none of them were so kind to have kept a catalog of the illnesses they found natives able to cure." This statement highlights that the Native Americans were highly skilled herbalists from an incredibly early time in history.

Traditional and Modern Uses of Herbal Medicine

Native Americans have always allied with plants in at least three ways: relationally, physically, and spiritually. This reciprocal relationship lays the foundation for how Indigenous peoples interact with plant remedies in what is now referred to as "herbalism." Herbalism for the First Peoples included a relationship with plants that allowed for an energetic exchange, which guided them on when and how to engage with the plant medicine. Sometimes this plant-human interaction would include a confirmation that the plant is needed for specific healing purposes; other times the plant could beckon to simply be examined and learned from. No matter the outcome, Native Americans historically have approached plants with

THE ROLES OF HEALERS IN NATIVE AMERICAN CULTURE

One of the most respected members of the tribe, the medicine healer was traditionally born into a lineage of healers or ordained through a dream or vision. Each healer always began their role as an apprentice for an extended amount of time and wasn't permitted to perform alone until each was deemed proficient in their skill. Like a priest, they would secure a connection with the "Creator" for the benefit of the community or individual. Traditional healers would employ different healing modalities such as drumming, chanting, praying, ceremony, purging, and plant and even animal substances. Some tools were symbolic, referring to the element that could bring the patient back into balance with the earth and Creator. One example is the feather, which symbolizes the element of air.

Healing ceremonies are sacred, usually done in medicine lodges, and considered closed to nontribal members. However, the healer can perform these ceremonies in the outdoors, if necessary. These acts of healing were one aspect of Native American healing that was forced underground or discontinued altogether out of fear or shame. In the seventeenth century, shamanism began to replace the medicine person or traditional healer, likely a desperate move to ward off the effects of colonization. The title "shaman" is often used in reference to Native American healers; however, this title is not of Native American origin but Siberian. It was later adopted into German *schamane*. Shamanism has historically been practiced in countries including Nepal, Mongolia, and China.

reverence because to do otherwise could lead to disharmony between the physical and spiritual body, manifesting as illness.

Sadly, until 1978, when the American Indian Religious Freedom Act was signed, Indigenous peoples didn't have the freedom to practice their traditional ways, including ceremonies and the use of herbs. This led to a lack of traditional knowledge passed down generationally. Meanwhile, during the 1960s and 1970s, herbalists of European descent were forming schools and authoring books using plant knowledge gleaned from Indigenous traditions. Many of these herbalists gained popularity and lucrative profits while Native Americans were still recovering and relearning their earth-based practices. It has taken perseverance for Native Americans to revive their traditional ways; however, because of this historic oppression, there remained a lack of Indigenous representation in herbalism until today.

The Medicine Wheel and the Four Directions

The Native American medicine wheel is a tool used to teach the human relationship to the natural world and how understanding the cyclical nature of life can help achieve intellectual, emotional, physical, and spiritual balance. The medicine wheel is separated into four equal parts, represented by a color, a plant, and a cardinal direction. Each part is connected further to a season (spring, summer, fall, or winter), a stage of life (infancy, adolescence, adulthood, or eldership), and an element (earth, air, water, or fire).

The cardinal directions are the starting point for understanding the rest of the layers. The sun rises in the east and is the first layer of the circle (represented by yellow), which correlates to spring, infancy, and the element of earth. The circle runs clockwise, making south the next quarter, symbolized by red and sharing a connection with summer, adolescence, and the air element or breath. Then there is west, which is black in color and associated with fall, adulthood, and the water element. The north, white like snow, symbolizes the winter phase, which is the time of eldership and is associated with the element of fire.

Within these circles are the lessons found in nature that provide guidance toward living a balanced life, which includes your innermost being and the animals, plants, and stones (minerals) surrounding you. The Lakota began referring to this acknowledgment of relatedness as "all my relations."

How Herbal Medicine Improves Health and Wellness

Herbal medicine is a complementary system of health care that may lessen your need to take part in allopathic medicine but should never take the place of medical care when necessary. The use of herbal medicine has many benefits, including nutritional support, restoration of body systems, and acute care for minor health challenges. Some people have even used plants to heal more complex health conditions, such as Lyme disease. However, if you are not collaborating with a trained professional, it is best to focus on how plants can ward off chronic disease within the body. Nutritionally speaking, many medicinal plants can be consumed through meals. Nettle leaves, which can be cooked in a soup, and burdock root, which is still a common food in Asian diets, were staples in the diets of the First Peoples. When using herbs to restore a system to homeostasis, we employ herbs that have an affinity for that system. One example is the well-known herb red raspberry leaf, which has long been associated with the reproductive system. Restorative herbs tone and strengthen the tissues and nerves within the system they are most aligned with. You may be familiar with this concept through the herb chamomile, which relaxes the nervous system.

Before the introduction of modern medicine, Native Americans looked toward plants to treat acute and chronic conditions. Today, many prescriptions mirror the constituents found in these plants. For example, aspirin, which is a medication synthesized from salicylic acid, has similarities to the chemical salicin, which is found in the bark of the white willow tree.

The Four Sacred Medicines

Each of the four sacred medicines is revered by all Native Americans, but they are bonded by the land and creation stories with specific tribes. For example, Californian tribes share the land where white sage grows. Cedar holds a space in the creation stories of the Navajo and Coast Salish peoples. The Potawatomi tell of how sweetgrass was one of the first plants smeared on the turtle's back by Sky Woman, the first woman to inhabit the earth. The sacred ally tobacco seems to permeate the traditions of all Native American tribes, but as a member of an eastern tribe, tobacco carries something even more special for me because I've heard stories of my ancestors harvesting this mighty plant.

The sacred medicines may share different lineages, but what they all have in common is that each one has been considered a generous giver to the Native American peoples and a gift from the Great Spirit. Cedar is revered for its large variety of uses, offering shelter, clothing, and a cleansing medicine. Sweetgrass is still cherished today for its purification abilities and resiliency in basketry. Tobacco is still prized in Indigenous communities and bartered with and given as gifts. White sage is considered a powerful ceremonial plant. When burned, the smoke from all the sacred plants can carry prayers to the Creator.

CEDAR

The cedar tree has historically always been a source of functionality to Indigenous peoples. They used its wood to create vessels, utensils, canoes, and homes. Because of its importance, it was often referred to as the "tree of life." Northwestern tribes use the large western red cedar to create intricate totem poles that symbolize their clan groups, commemorate their ancestors, or tell the stories of tribal legends or events of the past. Ceremonially, the twigs and flat leaves are burned to cleanse an area or person in the presence of illness. Historically, Native Americans attempted to treat smallpox with cedar, and research has confirmed that the essential oil thujone present in cedar kills airborne pathogens.

SAGE

Sage is a highly revered, sacred herb. Its smoke is strong, thick, and pungent, and like the dry heat produced in the depth of summer, it has a quality that ushers in an end to what has reached its full potential, cleansing and laying the foundation for new growth. Whereas sweetgrass brings in good energy, sage transforms the energy. Used before a ceremony, sage cleanses the spirit and the dwelling, creating a barrier between the ceremonial space and bad spirits. Additionally, science has confirmed desert sage has antioxidants that protect cells from environmental elements that cause infections.

SWEETGRASS

Sweetgrass is woven into baskets and Native American creation myths, such as the story of Sky Woman, which tells of how sweetgrass became one of the first plants of North America. The name is telling of its characteristics; sweetgrass has a vanilla-like aroma that is intensified when burned. Sweetgrass is traditionally braided and symbolic of the hair of Mother Earth—the three sections of the braid being mind, body, and soul—and braiding is done with a prayer of gratitude for Mother Earth's provisions. Sweetgrass is a powerful ceremonial plant and is burned with the intention of purifying the mind and ceremonial space.

TOBACCO

Tobacco was the first plant given to Indigenous peoples by the Creator and is the plant commonly offered as a gift of thankfulness to the sun each new day, to the earth when harvesting medicine, to the Creator after taking an animal's life, and to the water for its ability to sustain life. Tobacco is commonly used in ceremonies associated with birth, marriage, and death, as well as in personal prayer. This sacred plant is seen as a symbol of gratitude and is often carried in the medicine pouch of a traditionalist and can be burned in bundles, pipes, or cigars or simply thrown on a fire.

Healing Ceremonies in Native American Culture

Native American healing ceremonies are as connected to someone or something unworldly and powerful as prayers are in Abrahamic religions. Although intriguing to many people outside of the culture, Native American ways have historically been viewed as primitive, and efforts have been made to disconnect Indigenous peoples from their traditional ways and ceremonies.

Many eastern or first-contact tribes were decimated from the effects of colonization, and the ones that persevered were left with only remnants of their traditional ceremonial and plant knowledge—but fortunately they've had the wherewithal to revitalize their ways. Every tribe has endured its own story. Some were able to keep important facets of their unique traditional healing ceremonies and still practice them today; others took the knowledge of their peoples they still carried and began incorporating new aspects, sometimes from other tribes. In doing so, they revived traditional ways for the healing of their people. Revitalization is a process that is ongoing in many tribal communities, and the best way to honor it is to revere healing ceremonies but not seek to imitate them.

The Four Elements and Native American Spirituality

Most Indigenous peoples regard ceremonies as part of their private spiritual lives. I believe that Native American ceremonies should be looked upon with the wonder and respect that recognizes the strength of Native peoples to resist outside ways and hold on to the wisdom of their ancestors. The wisdom non-Indigenous people can adopt from healing ceremonies of Native Americans is how the power of the elements is woven into them to remind us of Creator's offerings. These elements of earth, air, water, and fire are recognized as healing modalities in Native American culture.

EARTH

The earth element is seen through the sweat-lodge ceremony that is done in a low dome-shaped shelter. This dome sometimes represents the womb of the mother, which grows new life just as the earth does. When we retreat into the earth for nourishment or ceremony, we become sedentary, drawing on her energy to renew our spirits. It is the intent that, when you go into a ceremony that reflects the nature of the earth element, you come out purified and reborn. This practice can be done through visualization. Plants that might be used in these ceremonies include sage and sweetgrass.

AIR

Smudging is the embodiment of the air element. Smudging is the practice of preparing or cleansing an item, person, or space for a traditional ceremony. It is believed that the smoke during a smudge ceremony moves through the air and can penetrate between the realms of creation, driving out negativity. Additionally, research has shown that the smoke of herbs can reduce airborne bacteria. The act of smudging is not exclusive to Indigenous culture; however, the sacred herbs mentioned in this book (cedar, sage, sweetgrass, and tobacco) have always belonged to the Native tribes that steward the land where they grow.

WATER

Without water, there is no life. We are born out of a womb full of water, and this element is cherished in the Native American culture for giving life. In sweat ceremonies, water is poured onto stones to produce steam that purifies and heals. Tribes such as the Blackfeet pass down stories of the realms of life and the sacredness of water; activists risk their lives to defend water resources not only for the people but also for the animals that are sustained by it. Water represents emotions and has the power to restore balance and harmony.

FIRE

An often-overlooked Native American ceremonial practice is storytelling. The telling of stories was traditionally done after the winter solstice when the plants and animals had retreated for the winter and nights sitting by a fire became long. Like the stories told by elders to the next generation, the fire acts as a messenger, penetrating other realms, allowing us to receive messages from Creator or ancestors passed. This element is part of the sacred pipe ceremony of the Lakota people and can just as easily be employed in your own personal ceremonies simply by lighting a candle or building a fire outdoors.

Types of Herbal Preparations

The way you choose to prepare your herbs will be decided by your skill level, resources, the amount of time you would like the herbal remedy to keep fresh before it expires, and what your desired effects are with the specific herb. To avoid overwhelming yourself, the best place to start is by infusing water with one herb; this is called a "simple," which allows you to experience the flavor, texture, and effect of the herb. For example, is the herb bitter, astringent, sweet, or sour? Does it dry your tongue or bring about moisture? As your skill level increases, decoctions may become the next obvious stepstone, or you may jump to infused oils because you wish for topical applications. Thankfully, herbs ease about the apothecary with grace, and the ones that prefer to be used in lesser quantities tend to make that obvious by their scent and flavor. Also, many of the herbs that would be best used by a trained herbalist are harder to access. An important consideration is whether to use dried herbs or fresh. For example, fresh herbs introduce water into oils, which can lead to bacterial growth. So, get creative, but be mindful of cleanliness and sanitation!

TEA

Infusing herbs into water, or making tea, may be the most emotionally supportive way to engage the nourishing benefits of plants. The act alone can bring you into the present moment, allowing for a pause at any time of the day. Making tea is simple; you combine boiled water (212°F) with your preferred herbs and allow the tea to steep for anywhere from two to twenty minutes. This process is usually done using more fragile plants such as flowers, leaves, and fruit. Infusing tools vary and include fillable disposable or reusable muslin tea bags, stainless steel tea infusers, French presses, and teapots with attached infusing baskets.

DECOCTION

A decoction is a method of boiling more tenacious plant materials, including barks, roots, nuts, and seeds, in water or another menstruum until up to half the liquid has evaporated, to fully extract the herb's medicinal benefits in heavier doses. Herbal decoctions have held a space in traditional and cultural plant medicine for thousands of years and sometimes even included minerals, stones, and parts of animals. To decoct herbs, add one teaspoon to one tablespoon of herb to one cup of water, and simmer while covered to maintain nutrients. You may also choose to remove the decoction from the heat and allow it to sit overnight before consuming.

TINCTURE

Due to its ability to extract a wide array of plant constituents, tincture-making is an amazingly effective method of creating plant remedies. To create a tincture, herbs are crushed and then macerated in a solvent such as alcohol, glycerin, or vinegar to create a pulp. The folk method of tincturing plants involves allowing the jarred maceration to sit in a dark place while shaking regularly for up to six weeks, then straining through a sieve and/or muslin or cheesecloth into a new container. Alcohol preserves the tincture longer, whereas glycerin and vinegar are best for children or those who avoid alcohol.

OILS AND SALVES

Herb-infused oils are often the first step to creating salves and can also be used in soapmaking. Traditionally, Native Americans would make a salve by combining animal fat with a strong herb decoction. Today, it is known that any presence of water allows for bacterial growth, and thus most people opt for an infused oil combined with a solid fat, such as coconut oil and beeswax. However, tallow is still known for its healing benefits. Creating infused herbal oils is like tincture-making because you macerate herbs in a solvent (in this case, an oil) for a desired length of time.

POULTICE

A poultice results from water boiled with aerial plant parts, roots, or both to create a thick paste that can be spread over the skin and covered with cloth, allowing the healing benefits of the plant to penetrate the skin. My grandmother used to mix cigarette tobacco with her saliva as a quick treatment for beestings! Although not very sophisticated, this mixture was a poultice. Traditionally, the herb would have been blended with a mucilaginous plant such as flax meal or slippery elm. The benefits of poultices include quelling local inflammation, decreasing swelling, and breaking sores such as boils.

Be Mindful of Herbal Dosage

Herb dosage varies from person to person and depends on the herb, the herbal preparation, and the health condition of the person being treated. The first step is to evaluate contraindications that would prohibit the consumption of a specific herb. For this, a valuable resource is a materia medica, a reference guide that lists how plants have been therapeutically used in the past. Successful herb-dosing also depends on body weight; a general guideline for tinctures is one drop per two pounds of body weight. For children, herbalists will use one of three methods: Clark's, Cowling's, or Young's Rule. The calculations for these can be easily found online. Also keep in mind that age can alter dosing, because as we grow older our liver function decreases.

Another method for adults is the titration method. To do this, the consumer will start at the lowest dose and increase gradually until the desired effects are felt. This method takes more time to integrate, but it can prevent the overconsumption of your herbal remedy. Additionally, if you experience a stronger reaction than preferred from taking an herb dosage, titrate down until you've achieved the desired effect. Last, if treating an acute condition, the herbal remedy is usually dosed in smaller amounts but more frequently throughout the day; for example, an herbal cough syrup would be given every two to three hours in teaspoon to tablespoon quantities. In the case of chronic conditions, the herbal preparation is more likely to be recommended in larger amounts but only one or two times per day. If needed, seek the guidance of a trained herbalist by contacting the American Herbalists Guild.

Respect the Gifts of the Earth

To carry an Indigenous mindset is to be intimately intertwined with the gifts offered by the earth. This way of life can and should be adopted by all groups of people to preserve our much-needed environmental resources. It is important to recognize that the way we treat the earth affects everyone currently alive and future generations to come. Involving children in practices that contribute to a healthier planet creates one of the greatest impacts. Activities can include teaching them the principles of recycling, how to choose more eco-conscious packaging, and how littering damages our lands and waterways.

Gardening is a therapeutic way to connect to the earth. Whether you engage in container gardening or you till a plot of soil, you will reap the rewards as you tend to the needs of your plants and are reminded of the effort it takes to grow nourishing and medicinal plants. Doing so will also increase your appreciation for the harvest you receive. An easy daily practice is to acknowledge how your basic need of hydration is met by the earth by saying a prayer to the water sourced from your home's pipes. Through this mindful act, you allow your relationship with the earth to become an intimate one and notice that even the smallest of details on earth are specially curated for you to have abundant life.

KEY TAKEAWAYS

Herbalism describes the interactive relationship between medicinal plants and humans. This relationship includes both spiritual and physical healing. It is still possible to honor the wisdom of Indigenous peoples by understanding their histories, listening to their stories, and respecting their boundaries during traditional ceremonies.

- Native American creation stories offer insights into the relationship Indigenous peoples have shared with plants. The relationship was deepened into knowledge systems as they worked with the plants and shared this wisdom with one another.

- The Native American medicine wheel offers a framework to help you live in intellectual, emotional, physical, and spiritual balance.

- The use of herbal medicine has many benefits, including nutritional support, restoration of body systems, and acute care for minor health challenges. More complex health conditions should always be supported by a trained professional.

- Dosages will be specific based on the preparation of the herbs and the herb used; reputable brands can offer insight, but, if necessary, locate a trained herbalist through groups like the American Herbalists Guild for in-depth assistance.

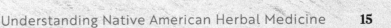

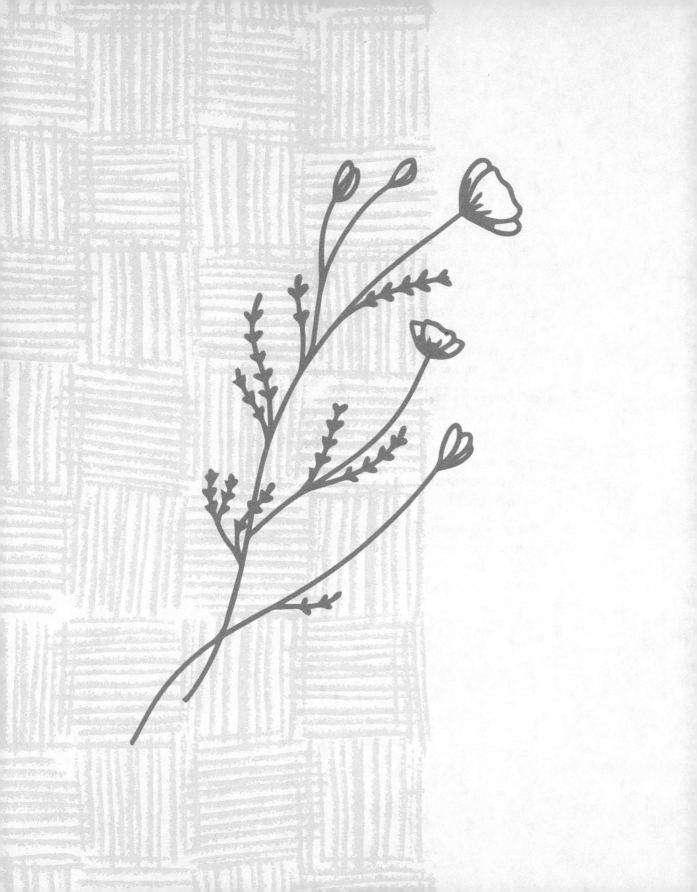

Preparing Your Tools and Ingredients

In this chapter, you will learn about the aspects of gathering plants from the wild as well as from a garden. More than just obtaining medicinal herbs, this process of collecting your own plant medicines is an act of building a plant-human relationship that will support you in becoming a more well-rounded herbalist. You'll sharpen your skills of examining crucial details of a plant and its environment to ensure safety and develop the wisdom to slow down when unsure before disturbing the ecosystem. You will also learn what tools you may need, how and when to harvest, and how best to do so while leaving the plant to thrive. Interaction with plants and herbalism also comes with the joy of connecting with other plant enthusiasts in your community, which is often done through procurement of rare herbs or herb seedlings. Last, you'll learn to tend to the fruits of your labor by drying and storing your harvests for health benefits all year long.

Learn to Identify Medicinal Plants and Herbs

Important reasons to be certain you're harvesting the correct plant include: to avoid toxic plants, to ensure you're harvesting the correct plant for the corresponding medicinal need, and to avoid harvesting endangered or threatened species. Characteristics such as leaf shape, stem shape, size, flower, color, and aroma all aid in helping identify a safe medicinal plant or garden plant species. Because plants only flower at specific times of year and some only biennially, leaf identification is more imperative. The more characteristics you can identify about the plant, the more confident you will feel before harvesting a plant for medicinal purposes while avoiding safety mishaps.

You can learn more about endangered or threatened species through United Plant Savers. These species are usually those that grow only in specific regions or conditions and have been highly desirable, typically for commercial reasons. Two examples include white sage and goldenseal root. White sage is a medicinal herb that is important to Native communities of California and is often overharvested to create commercialized smudging products. Goldenseal root is threatened due to the loss of its natural habitat and illegal poaching. Additionally, medicinal roots take three to five years to regenerate, and overharvesting inhibits the regrowth process. Being aware of these types of plant-cultural connections, growing conditions, and habits are ways to honor Native American traditions. These lessons can also be applied when sourcing dried herbs; it is important to know who harvested the plant and if it was done with intention and care.

The Art of Wildcrafting

Wildcrafting is the practice of gathering plants from their natural habitats in a way that is ethical and sustainable. This act becomes an experience of intimately acknowledging the plant, the ecosystem, and the traditional lands of the Indigenous group that have historically lived there. The first step is to learn how to properly identify the plants you are harvesting. For this step, a forager's field guide for the specific region you are harvesting is a wise investment. It is also helpful to take note of the habitat to help you determine if the plant is one that would thrive there. Is it shady, sunny, moist, or dry? Checking off these factors will allow you to feel more confident that you have chosen the correct medicinal specimen.

If you're still in an early learning stage, begin with easy-to-find weeds, such as dandelion and plantain, to build your confidence.

After you've determined the plant is correctly identified, approach the plant holistically, considering factors such as where its energy is focused, its current phase of life, how it reproduces (through rhizome or seed), and when it produces seeds. If the plant is going to seed, it is best practice to spread as many seeds onto the ground as possible. If you're harvesting roots in the fall, leave some of the root for regrowth. Avoid overharvesting. Only harvest what you need and will use in your personal medicine-making or creations for your community.

Important Tools for Foraging

Most hobbies require the use of tools. However, when it comes to working with plants, do not let a lack of tools become a barrier. Depending on the medicinal herb you are intending to harvest, you may need little more than your fingers or a stick. This is especially true when harvesting with children; my daughter's favorite herb to collect is violets, and we often simply pluck the dainty flowers off with our fingers, but she also sometimes enjoys using her childproof scissors. I have also dug up dandelion roots with a stick and my hands. Although this job is one that could be made more efficient with more intricate tools, they are not always necessary. However, if you have reached the stage in your herbal journey in which professional tools are needed, you may want to start with a foraging pouch to carry your tools so they don't get misplaced or forgotten while you're out playing in the dirt. Tools are a financial investment, and a few popular items are described in this section. Many herbalists and gardeners have preferences on brands of equipment and are usually happy to share their knowledge.

A BRUSH

When harvesting roots, expect to get dirt under your nails (unless you choose to wear gloves), but I recommend you allow the nutrients of the rich soil to cover your hands. According to a study named "The Farm Effect," beneficial bacteria found in soil can boost your respiratory and gut health and even release dopamine, making you happier. Of course, you'll want to wash those roots before making medicine, so a good sturdy, bristled brush (preferably with natural bristles) is helpful to clean dirt within the cracks and crevices of your root harvests. Wash your harvest under flowing water until the water running out the bottom is clear.

A KNIFE

A lightweight knife will sufficiently harvest most smaller wildflowers, leaves, or mushrooms. However, when foraging transitions into a substantial hobby, it may be time to invest in a high-quality stainless steel knife to aid in unearthing deeper roots such as burdock, chicory, or dandelion. These knives can also be used to break up soil and pull medium plants out of the ground. Many trained herbalists suggest the Japanese garden knife sold under the name "hori hori." Regardless of the brand, an exceptionally durable knife is needed to hold up to multiple tasks such as digging, splitting transplants, sawing, and weeding.

SCISSORS OR PRUNERS

Scissors are necessary for harvesting tender aerial parts of herbs, whereas pruners are best for hardier-stemmed plants, but the reach of their blade is limited. Pruners offer a clean cut to the woodier stems should you need to harvest them, which will prevent disease from invading the plant. Never break hardier-stemmed plants because you may expose them to insect infestations or disease. When choosing a pair of pruners, consider they are going to be one of the most useful tools you carry and worth the investment. Be sure to look for a pair that fits comfortably in your hand.

GATHERING BASKETS

I have gone on my share of foraging trips with just a simple paper bag for transporting my harvest, but a beautiful gathering basket has the magic of making the occasion feel more special. Baskets come in all shapes, sizes, and levels of quality, ranging from a thrift-shop find to a handcrafted woven basket. Herbal conferences or artisan markets are a wonderful place to buy baskets you can treasure for years. The practical benefit of baskets is they allow air to move all around the plant, preventing mold from growing.

Carefully Select Your Gathering Site

Before gathering plants, it is imperative that you gather the knowledge necessary to wildcraft responsibly. You can do so by seeking out resources such as a local tribe, your county extension office, or a trained wildcrafter in your area. You may choose to start by deciding what plant you'd like to harvest, becoming familiar with its natural habitat, and seeking out that space. Or you can decide on a gathering location and harvest what is available there.

When choosing a gathering location, first ensure you are not harvesting on private or protected property. Be sure to check your local laws about collecting on public lands. You'll then want to assess if there is any contamination, such as fumes from passing vehicles; a potentially contaminated water source close by; harmful insect infestations; or the presence of pesticides, fungicides, or both. Otherwise, you could be unintentionally taking in harmful chemicals. You'll also want to make sure the area has not experienced any stress, creating fragility within the plant community. Examples include a recent flooding or disruption from construction.

Observe the quantity of plants available, and never harvest more than you can use; a good rule of thumb is to not harvest more than 5 percent of the plant population. Sometimes you will find that one area is sparse in the desired plant, but if you walk a few more feet, you'll find a more abundant stand ready to be harvested. As an ethical wildcrafter, your role is to ensure that the plants continue to thrive and proliferate by supporting their space within the habitat.

Tips for Harvesting Plants and Herbs

Once you experience the pleasure of using freshly harvested herbs, you will find it difficult to switch back to store-bought dried herbs. Watching the plant evolve throughout the year by growing it yourself and tending to its needs throughout the season, or by visiting the location where it grows and caring for its natural habitat, opens you up to a more in-depth experience of the natural world. If you start to feel overwhelmed in the garden, invite friends and neighbors over for a harvesting party or to try recipes for preserving the herbs. Later in this book, you will learn the benefits of drying your herbs, but some herbs such as basil can also be preserved in oils that can be used in cooking and frozen into cubes for later use.

The following list breaks down the separate parts of the plants and guides you through the process of harvesting them for immediate use or preservation. These tips apply to your garden herbs or while foraging medicinal plants.

ABOVEGROUND PLANTS

Mornings are the best time to harvest the aerial parts of the plant—the stem, leaves, and flowers—all parts of the plant that receive air, excluding the bark. Harvesting aerial parts takes little more than sharp, clean scissors or a knife. Remember that a clean cut is best to avoid making the plant vulnerable to fungus or insects. Depending on the plant, you'll likely want to harvest the entire stem; this is done by working your way down until you find a spot where two sets of new leaves are growing. Just above this intersection is where you cut. Doing so will also encourage bushier growth and a healthier plant.

ROOTS

The energy of the plant is focused back into the earth in the fall, making it the ideal time of year to harvest roots. This task takes more skill and hardier equipment such as a strong garden spade, a digging stick, and/or pruners. Your goal is to loosen the dirt around the root as much as possible, allowing you to cleanly remove the root once you get to the end. Be prepared for roots to grow twelve or more inches deep, such as in the case of burdock roots. It is best to be mindful not to overdisturb the ground and to replace soil after you've harvested your medicinal root.

BARK

Fall is also the season for harvesting bark. However, when first starting out, always go with a trained wildcrafter because if you don't harvest bark correctly, the tree may not survive. According to Juliette Carr from Old Ways Herbal, "Trees are keystone species, meaning they form the center of the complex ecological web that surrounds them"—therefore, harvesting from them should be done with care. The bark of the tree is always interacting with the world around it, shifting its compounds to withstand the surroundings. It is through this process that the desired medicinal constituents are formed.

FRUITS AND SEEDS

Late summer is the time to harvest fruits and seeds. Berries appear after the plant has flowered for the season. The most prominent medicinal berries include elderberry, hawthorn, and rose hip. Then there are the nutritional berries such as blackberries, raspberries, and huckleberries. Before harvesting berries, you'll want to look for a rich pigment to make sure they are fully ripe; by that point, they are likely easy to pop off or shake from the stem. It's also important to be 100 percent certain in your plant identification because some berries may contain toxic compounds. Without certainty, it is best to let the plant be.

HOW TO SOURCE RARE HERBS

Sourcing hard-to-find plants and herbs can take a little extra time and effort but is a task that can take you on a fun journey and allow you to connect with fellow plant enthusiasts. The first place you can start is by visiting a local health-food store; you may be amazed at the amount of herb jars they have in their bulk-herb sections, which allow you to buy dried culinary and medicinal herbs by the ounce, saving you money. The jars are usually arranged in alphabetical order so you can easily find the one you are looking for. If the store does not carry your preferred herb, the staff can sometimes place a special order for it, suggest a resource for buying it, or offer a substitute. In a pinch, having an understanding of what body system the herb supports will help you find an alternative option.

Sourcing live plants may be a larger hurdle but can also lead you to some fun places. I love visiting plant and herb festivals or conferences. These events connect you with growers who are enthusiastic and will be excited to share their tips. These herb farmers typically also harvest and dry herbs on their farms, selling them at markets or online. Purchasing herbs that have been dried in the same vicinity of where they were grown and haven't spent time on a retail shelf will offer you a superior herb full of medicinal value. Once you find these high-quality herbs, you will become more critical about where you purchase your herbs.

Gather with Patience and Intention

Part of the plant-human interaction is to respect the plant's boundaries, asking permission before harvesting; through this practice, our listening skills become enhanced and we cultivate a deeper relationship to our intuition. If permission is granted, it is a best practice to offer a sacrifice; for the Indigenous, it may be tobacco, but you are allowed to create your own offering—if it is environmentally friendly, of course. Suggestions include a stone, cornmeal, water, a piece of hair, a song, or a prayer. Don't worry if it is not perfect; the goal is to acknowledge the sacrifice the plant is making for you in that you are also recognizing its livelihood.

Growing Your Own Herb Garden

Growing your own herb garden is probably easier than you think! Herbs are such gracious plants; many tolerate less favorable conditions compared to many vegetables. Before installing your herb garden, it is important to look over your landscape for wet and dry areas and sunlight exposure, because most herbs prefer a sunny location with well-drained soil. Some herb gardeners even choose to blend herbs into their landscapes, which works exceptionally well for most medicinal herbs and adds to the beauty of your living space. Other options include aboveground gardens or medicine-wheel-themed gardens, but if space is limited, remember many herbs (like calendula) can be grown in pots and still supply you with a modest harvest. No matter your method, tending these plants will expand your plant knowledge and support your physical and emotional health.

Soil health should be a focus. Sometimes it seems obvious that your soil is rich, but if you question your soil's health, collect a sample, and take it to your local agricultural center for an evaluation so they can suggest amendments. You'll also want to choose between starting from seed or purchasing plants. My method for choosing between seeds and plants is to learn about the success of germination per seed; if it is an easy to moderate seed to germinate, I opt for seeds, but if not, seedlings or plants, although more expensive, offer greater security that you'll get a harvest that year. Also consider the time it takes for the seed to reach maturity, and be sure you have an ample window of time; if not, then seedlings may be the best option.

The Benefits of Drying Herbs and Plants

Our Indigenous and European ancestors employed many ways to preserve yearly harvests, such as infusing medicinal plants in alcohol, vinegar, or oil/fat. Although these methods have benefits for specific circumstances, they require more space, time, and effort. The simplest way to preserve your harvest is to dry or dehydrate your plants, which is the process of removing all the moisture from the plant to safely store it without mold growing. Dehydrating herbs also offers the benefit of having them at hand and ready to be used in future herbal preparations. The absolute least expensive way to dry plants is to hang them upside down in a well-ventilated, dark spot indoors or other space with limited humidity. Or you can also use your oven on the lowest temperature to speed up the drying process, and if budget allows, a dehydrator can be purchased. It is not essential that you buy an expensive dehydrator, because the low-budget ones often can be sufficient for herbs. I have found that plants such as passionflower that have thicker watery stems are not as easy to dry at home, so I simply remove the leaves and flowers from the vine. However, the thin stems found in the mint family can be dried along with the leaves, and you can crumble the leaves in with the stems or remove the leaves from stems. Depending on the size of your harvest, you will have enough dried herbs to last you until the next harvesting season, saving you money and offering you a more flavorful herb experience.

Best Storage Practices

My guess is your goal is to have enough herbs to last you a year until your next opportunity to freshly harvest again. In that case, it is vital that you learn how to store your dried herbs safely. However, this area can be one of great frustration for even the experienced herb preserver. The most common mistake is storing the herbs before they are completely dehydrated, which leads to bacteria and mold growth within the container. Even just a couple of leaves not dried fully can destroy an entire batch, so if you live in a humid environment, this hazard is something to pay extra attention to. Once you have determined the leaves are fully dried, a glass jar is usually the most ideal storage container, but jars do need more space, so you can also try a vacuum-sealed food-storage bag. You can also order Mylar bags for food storage and order moisture and oxygen absorbers for added safety. Remember, oxygen and moisture are not your friends when it comes to storing dried herbs. Last, always make sure your dried plants are not being exposed to excess light. Although it is beautiful to display your dried herbs, it is not always practical, because the light exposure will decrease their color and vitality. This process requires trial and error to learn, so do not take it too hard if a batch does not survive; just compost it and move on, knowing you will get better each year.

KEY TAKEAWAYS

Harvesting your own medicinal plants, either by cultivation or foraging for them in their natural habitats, is rewarding and economically advantageous. The act of gathering plants aligns you with the seasons and has a positive impact on mental and emotional health.

- To avoid toxic plants and endangered or threatened species, characteristics such as leaf and stem shape and size and flower color or aroma aid in identifying a safe medicinal-plant or garden-plant species.

- Careful selection of a gathering site takes being aware of the property and contamination status, the condition of the plants you're aiming to harvest, and the density of the population to ensure there is enough present to harvest without overharvesting.

- Gathering plants with patience and intention includes asking the plant for permission and cultivating the intuition within us to receive confirmation from the plants.

- Growing an herb garden not only offers you more vibrant medicinal plants to work with but also has a positive impact on your spiritual, emotional, and physical health.

- Drying herbs is the most cost-effective and space-saving way to store your seasonal harvest to use throughout the year. Storage options vary, and the deciding factor is usually based on space and financial investment.

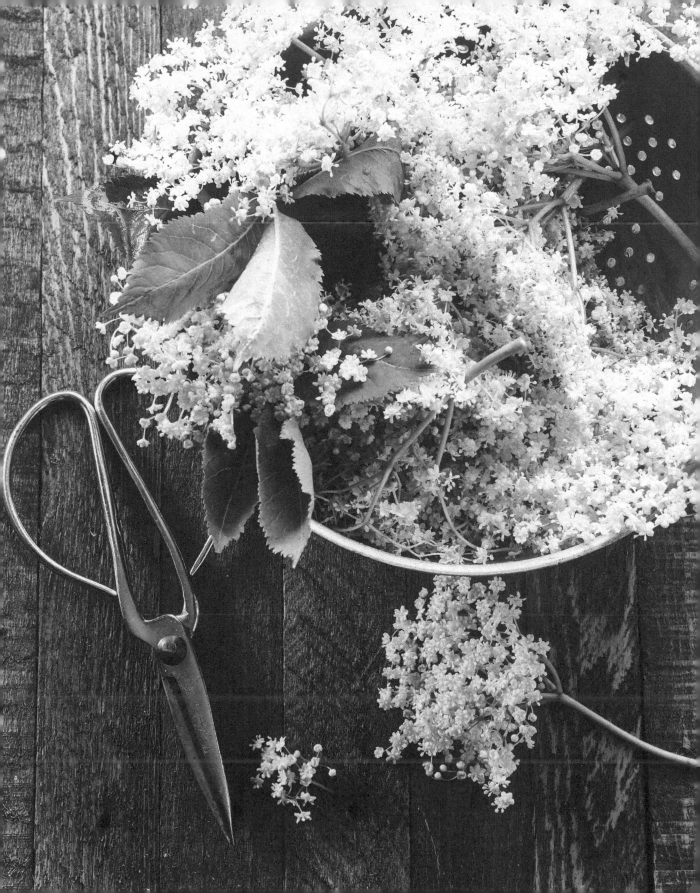

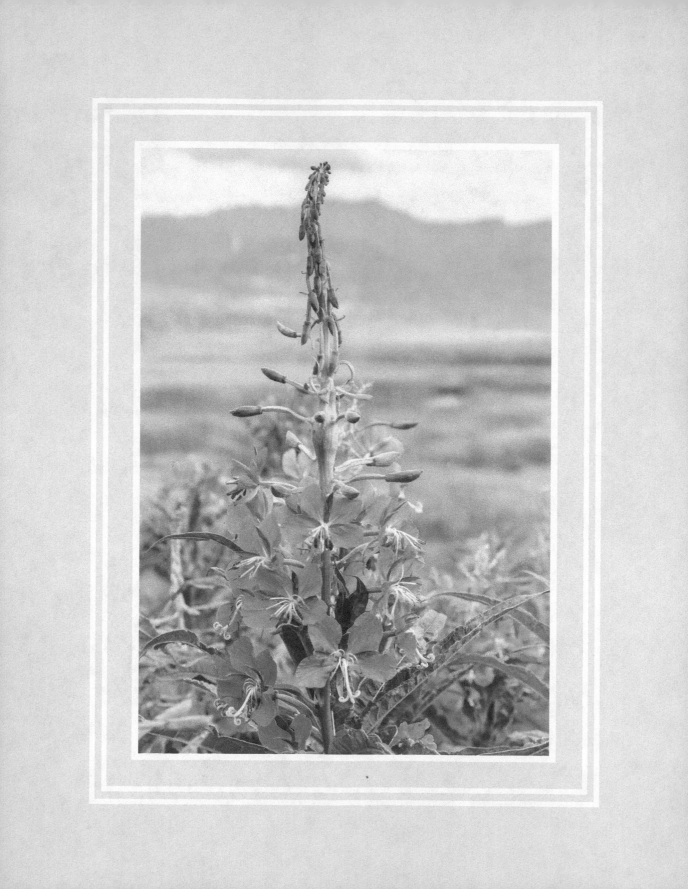

PART II

Essential Herbs to Know

In this part, you will explore nearly thirty medicinal plants that the Native Americans historically used. Each profile will give you information on the geographical location where the plant can be located, the landscape it prefers to grow in, how to identify it by distinguishing factors, and tips on harvesting the plant. You will learn about how the plant has been historically used by Native Americans and how it is used today. It is important to remember there are still Native Americans using these plants in traditional ways and passing this knowledge down to future generations.

Deciding which plants to include in this section was difficult. I chose to focus mostly on plants native to the North American continent with a couple exceptions. This excluded some popular plants, such as mullein and hawthorn, even though Native tribes did eventually learn of their benefits from Europeans and currently include them in their healing practices. To my knowledge, each plant can be wildcrafted if you have the capability, and most can easily be purchased in dried form online or in retail establishments. The plants are listed in alphabetical order by only their common names, but learning their botanical names can offer you more insight into the varied species available in your specific area.

Anise Hyssop

Parts used: *leaves, stems, flowers*

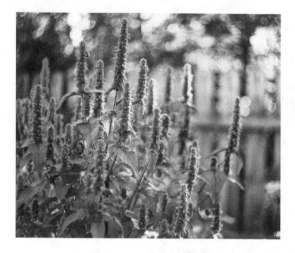

Anise hyssop is a member of the mint family, so its characteristics include a square stem; paired, heart-shaped, and serrated leaves; and tubular flowers that are pink to purple and hairy. Herbs in the mint family are aromatic, and when hyssop is crushed, the leaves emit a sweet, licorice-like aroma. Hyssop grows in sunny prairies and can be cultivated easily in a sunny spot in the ground. Dead-heading, or cutting plants just below a set of two leaves, early in the season encourages new growth and a bushier plant. Full harvesting can be done once the plant flowers two to three inches. Hyssop can be used fresh or can be dried to add into tea blends for colds and digestive support. It could also be used as a steam, tea, or wash.

Native Americans used hyssop as a respiratory aid and to reduce fever. The Cheyenne created cold infusions with the leaves of hyssop to comfort chest pain from coughing and as a cold remedy. The Haudenosaunee created a wash with hyssop to treat poison ivy and itch. Poultices of hyssop leaves and flowers were also placed on swollen areas for relief. Ceremonially, the Cree included these beautiful flowers in medicine bundles, believing the plant offered protection from evil spirits. Medicine bundles are different from medicine bags; a bundle would be one or more plants wrapped and held together by a string in a "bundle" and used in a smoke ceremony; medicine bags are leather pouches worn around the neck or waist that carry medicinal herbs.

Black Cohosh

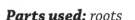

Parts used: *roots*

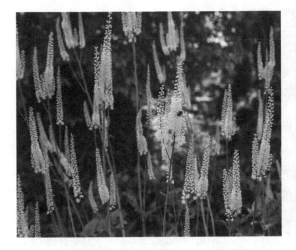

Cohosh, the Algonquin word for "gnarly" or "rough," refers to the root, the part of this herb that is used medicinally. Black cohosh blooms from June to September and has small, white, petalless flowers protruding up like a wand or spire. Because of this, black cohosh is sometimes referred to as "fairy candle." However, other folk names of the medicinal root include "black snakeroot" and "black bugbane." A woodland plant, black cohosh can be found south of Maine and westward through Missouri. It prefers shaded areas with good moisture retention. Black cohosh plants reproduce through the seed and rhizomes. The seeds have a low germination rate and need stratification (exposure to warm temperatures followed by cold) to germinate successfully. To support the reproduction of black cohosh, spread the seeds, leave a partial amount of the root, and only harvest plants at least three years old.

A poultice of this root was used by some tribes to treat snakebites, and it was used as a tea to treat colds, coughs, constipation, rheumatism, fatigue, hives, and pain. Black cohosh is best known for its ability to balance hormones and is recommended for menopausal symptoms. I can't help but notice the symbolism of the beautiful feminine flowers being the identifying element of this flower and the black root being the medicinal part, which in my mind reflects the growing dormancy of the womb. Black cohosh is also recommended by herbalists for other female reproductive disorders such as PCOS, fibroids, and PMS.

Black Haw

Parts used: *bark*

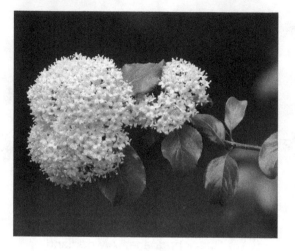

Black haw belongs to the honeysuckle family. You can find this bushy shrub, which grows to a height of ten to twenty-five feet, in dry woods and thickets and on rocky hillsides in fertile soil in states east of Texas, except for Florida. It has dark green leaves and clusters of small white flowers that bloom in early summer. Black haw also features small, black, edible berries that are extremely sweet and can be used to create a natural dye. Historically, black haw has had an affinity for all aspects of women's health. According to James A. Duke, author of *The Green Pharmacy*, black haw (also called cramp bark) has at least four compounds that help relax the uterine muscles, decreasing menstrual cramps as well as other muscle spasms.

Additionally, it has been called upon to support every aspect of pregnancy, including the prevention of morning sickness and miscarriage, reducing pain during childbirth, and even easing the recovery process after giving birth. I strongly suggest seeking the advice of a trained professional before using any herb during pregnancy. Native Americans knew of black haw's ability to induce labor, and it was administered during childbirth to promote a quicker birth and afterward to strengthen the reproductive organs. Black haw is also useful as a kidney stimulant and for urinary conditions, acting as a diuretic. Black haw cleanses the kidneys, preventing water retention.

Boneset

Parts used: *leaves, flowers*

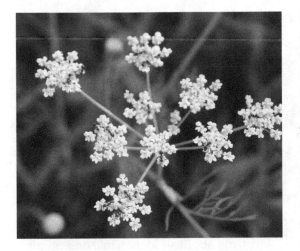

Boneset is native to North America and found in marshlands and meadows in states east of the Dakotas. It reaches up to five feet in height and has a hairy stem with opposite-pointed leaves united at the base. The leaves are oblong and pointed, and from July to October, the flat-topped flower heads bloom. According to the website Henriette's Herbal, boneset "deserves to be esteemed as one of the most useful medicines of the people." It's an intensely bitter herb, which supports the liver by increasing gastric juices. Boneset is almost completely relaxing with very little stimulating properties, so when formulating herbal remedies with this plant, it is helpful to add a stimulating herb such as ginger or cinnamon. Boneset works slowly but steadily; however, unlike a tonic herb, it shouldn't be taken for longer than six months at a time, and it is wise to research contraindications with prescriptions.

Native Americans used boneset to treat dengue fever, a mosquito-borne illness also referred to as "breakbone fever." Several tribes such as the Menominee and Cherokee tribes have a history of creating a strong tea with boneset to treat colds, fever, and the pain from arthritis and rheumatism. The root was used by the Mesquakies to treat snakebite wounds. Also referred to as "feverwort," boneset has the ability to break a fever. Boneset was the plant remedy used in the most extreme of cases, such as during flu epidemics. C. J. Hemple, a nineteenth-century physician, noted the herb that "relieved the disease . . . was familiarly called boneset."

Burdock

Parts used: *roots, tender leaves*

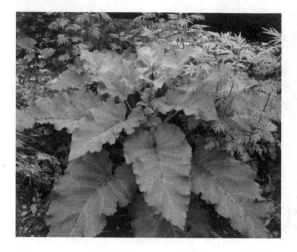

Burdock is a biennial plant, meaning it flowers and produces seeds on its second year before perishing. Because of this aspect, it is best to harvest this root on its second year and in late fall, but first-year roots are also edible. First-year plants have no stem, and they grow in a basal formation, meaning they arise directly from the ground. In the second year, burdock grows a stem that is about six inches tall, and purple flowers will protrude from the plant's head. There are at least ten different species of burdock found throughout the whole North American continent, growing in rocky soils, abandoned lots, fields, roadsides, and other disturbed places. Due to their rocky habitats, digging them up can be a chore, and the root usually breaks off ten to fifteen inches down. Newer leaves that are soft and tender can be boiled and eaten, and the root is a staple in Asian cuisines.

Historically, burdock root has been considered a blood purifier. The Menominee and Micmac Tribes used burdock root for skin sores, and the Cherokee, Delaware, and Haudenosaunee used it for rheumatism. Writer Michelle Loftis accounted how "Cowlitz Indians call this herb '*tcuktcu'k*,' and the Skagit Indians call it '*xexe'bats*' saying it came with the whites in hayseed, thereby seeming to place its origin with early settlers. Translated, it seems to mean the same thing, which is 'sticks to everything.'" That didn't stop the Cowlitz Tribe as well as the Chippewa from using it for whooping cough. Tribes also used burdock root topically for healing skin sores.

California Poppy

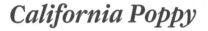

Parts used: *flowers, leaves, roots*

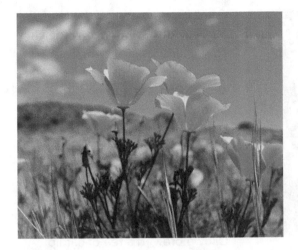

The state flower of California, the California poppy is an enchanting flower that grows in open meadows and can be cultivated in most states; however, it is native to California, Oregon, Washington, Nevada, and Arizona. Poppies are drought-tolerant and prefer sandy soil and full sun. The flowers are yellow to bright orange and are very delicate; the four petals of the flower close in the evenings and when it's chilly outside, and they'll likely fall from the plant once picked. California poppy's foliage is unique, fernlike, and silvery-green in color. All parts of California poppy can be used as medicine, and the leaves were boiled and eaten as food by Native Americans. They're simple to harvest, either by cleanly cutting the aerial parts you need or by pulling up the shallow root whole.

California poppy is considered an analgesic and sedative. Californian tribes used poppy as a toothache remedy, and the juice from the root would have been washed over the head to quell pain and over lactating breasts to stop milk production. The juice was also consumed for stomachaches. California poppy is currently used for sleeplessness and pediatric bed-wetting; the Natives knew of these uses, and instead of having the child take in the medicine internally, they would place the flower under the child's pillows for it to work on an energetic level. California poppy is not considered an opiate or addictive; it may have some of the same effects as the opium poppy but to a lesser degree.

Catnip

Parts used: *stems, leaves, flowers*

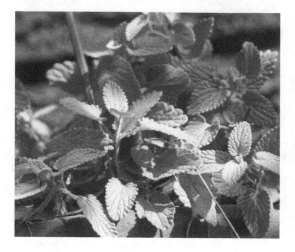

Catnip is a member of the mint family and shares those identifying characteristics including a square stem, simple opposite leaves, and strong aromatic qualities. The most potent medicine comes from the leaves and flowering tops (which are dainty with a grayish pink hue) that bloom between July and August. According to Wendy Makoons Geniusz, author of *Our Knowledge Is Not Primitive*, the Ojibwe brewed a tea of catnip leaves to purify the blood when consumed, and patients with cold or flu symptoms are soaked in an infusion of the herb to raise the body temperature, causing the fever to break. Research has confirmed the efficacy of this usage in addition to catnip's usefulness in relieving colds, upper respiratory infections, and congestion.

Eastern tribes blended catnip with a variety of other herbs in a syrup to reduce coughing and "prescribed" the tea for intestinal cramps and gas. Additionally, Lumbee folk healers would create a topical application including self-heal, fever grass, and catnip to heal skin wounds. Catnip tea has always been considered a very safe medicinal herb to treat children, and the Delaware, Hoh, and Haudenosaunee peoples employed this herb often for colicky infants or when children would complain about stomachaches or sleeplessness. These uses all highlight catnip's ability to relax smooth muscles, including uterine muscles in the case of menstrual cramps. Additionally, the Cherokee considered catnip to be a strengthening tonic; in herbalism, a tonic herb is believed to enhance the function of specific tissues, so in this case, catnip strengthens the digestive and nervous systems.

Cattail

Parts used: *roots, leaves, stems, flower, pollen, sap*

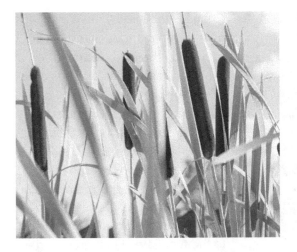

Supplying safe cover for deer and den material for the *wazhushk* (meaning "muskrat" in Ojibwe), cattails are as useful for the animal kingdom as they have been for the Native Americans. Despite the belief that cattails are an invasive species, they are one of the most versatile wild plants. Cattails are mucilaginous plants, meaning they have a gelatinous texture. They are water-loving and grow along thickets, marshes, moist fields, and wetlands. The plants are recognized by their thin, sturdy stalks that end with a brown cigar-shaped head called a candlewick. This is another plant that offers nutritious, medicinal, and household benefits. Parts of cattails are used in basketry and to fashion mats, and the candlewick (which doesn't retain water) can be used for insulation.

The entire plant is edible, and all parts offer digestive support. The young stems can be consumed raw or boiled, the lower part of the leaves can be used in salads, and the candlewick of the cattail can be roasted. Even the sap and pollen from it is useful as a thickening agent in stews, similar to cornstarch. The pollen can also be added to baking mixes for nutritional support. Medicinally, cattail pollen is astringent (tightens and restricts tissues), helping control bleeding. The root was used as a poultice on infections, blisters, stings, and infections. Internally, cattails were used for abdominal cramps and coughs. Between the leaves of a cattail plant, you'll find a jelly that can be applied topically and ingested for antiseptic benefits and to relieve pain and inflammation.

Chaga Fungi

Parts used: *fruiting body*

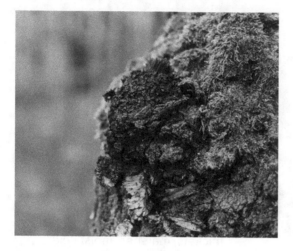

Chaga is technically not a plant. It's a fungus that appears as a solid growth on the side of birch trees. It is nutritionally dense and has a history with humanity that goes back thousands of years. Chaga supports the continued life of the birch tree, which is widespread throughout the Northern Hemisphere and is the host of the chaga's mycelial mass. Meanwhile, the birch tree transfers its medicinal properties to the fungi, helping it grow larger. Chaga is usually found on birch trees that are at least forty years old, and the fungi take five to ten years to fully form. In recent years, the overharvesting of chaga for its commercial use has left these fungi in danger, which means it could also lead to the vulnerability of the birch tree. So, although viewing chaga in its natural habitat can be rewarding, it is best to buy sustainably cultivated chaga rather than harvesting it yourself.

Canadian tribes such as the Cree, the Ojibwe, and the Denesuliné peoples use chaga to treat ailments such as tuberculosis, stomach ulcers, joint pain, and even rheumatic pain. Chaga is recognized now for its potent antioxidant benefits stimulating our immune system, reducing inflammation, blood pressure, and cholesterol. Chaga is complementary to coffee and can be added to your coffee beverage or used on its own; the flavor is earthy with hints of vanilla. Due to the woody texture, it is not edible as a food itself, but it can be sprinkled on foods in powdered form.

Chokecherry

Parts used: *berries*

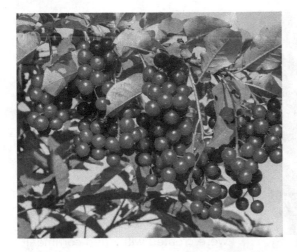

Chokecherry was such a staple in the diets of the Cheyenne and Blackfoot peoples that they simply referred to this plant as "berry" in their native tongues. A member of the rose family, this deciduous bush grows abundantly throughout North America and can be consumed raw or cooked. Nutritionally, chokecherries are high in vitamin C (boosting immunity), manganese (which supports the thyroid), cell-protecting compounds called antioxidants, and other disease-preventing phytonutrients. As a wild edible, chokecherry can be juiced, made into jellies and syrups, and even fermented to create fizzy beverages. Medicinally, chokecherries can be used to treat several ailments, including anxiety, the common cold, stomach distress, and other digestive complaints. According to the book *A Treasury of American Indian Herbs*, powdered chokecherry was also smoked like tobacco as a remedy for head colds.

Chokecherries are a rewarding plant to forage because they are so abundant and delicious. They can be found in open woodlands or on rocky terrain and prefer partially sunny areas. The chokecherry shrub blooms dense clusters of white flowers that move outward like a cone, and in the spring and in late summer, chokecherry fruit ripen in clusters. The toxic look-alike to chokecherries is buckthorn, which don't grow in clusters and have thorns, whereas the chokecherry doesn't. The leaves are two to four inches long, are oblong to nearly oval, and grow alternately on the two sides of the stem. It is easier to spot chokecherries when they are not fully ripened and are bright red. So, take note of their location and return to harvest them before the birds decide to.

Corn

Parts used: *kernels, stalk, silk, husk*

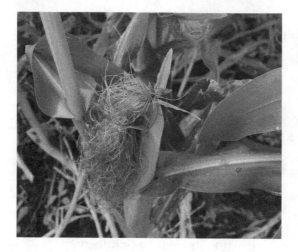

Corn is featured in the Tuscarora legend "The Corn Spirit," in which villagers had an awakening when they took their abundant corn harvests for granted and a man named Dayohagwenda delivered the dire message to his people that the corn spirit was saddened. Corn has always been held in high esteem by Native Americans. Just as medicinal as it is nutritious, corn was used in many forms: Poultices were created with dried cornmeal and applied to skin burns, swelling, and ulcers; and corn oil could be used to calm eczema and dry skin. The skin was also exposed to the smoke of the burned cob to stop the itch and irritation from insect bites.

Corn silk is still commonplace today in herbalism. Dried or fresh corn silk can be brewed into a tea. It has an affinity for the kidneys and bladder, releasing excess retained water, which can decrease blood pressure. Nutritionally, corn is high in several B vitamins, which support milk flow for nursing mothers. In true Native form, nothing was ever wasted, and even the husk of the corn was used in the making of baskets, sleeping mats, rattling sticks, and the still-adored corn-husk doll. Spiritually, corn is offered as a sacrifice to the spirit when harvesting and in traditional ceremonies. Corn remains a mainstay in many medicine cabinets in the form of cornstarch, body powders, and even dry shampoos.

Cotton Root

Parts used: *bark of the root*

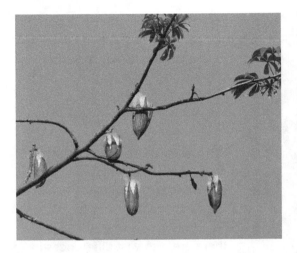

The bark of the cotton root is the herbal opposite of black haw in matters of pregnancy; whereas black haw aids in reducing the chance of spontaneous abortion, cotton root is an abortifacient. In her book *The Natural Pregnancy Book*, Aviva Romm states, "Cotton root bark is reliable for safely and gently promoting contractions." Cotton root can also bring on menstruation as well as treat endometriosis. Also, due to the stimulating properties of cotton root, it has been used as an aphrodisiac, intensifying orgasms.

Cotton root is a medicinal plant that tells a story of the similarities of African and Native American herbalists. Like the Native Americans, Africans have a long history of using plants for medicinal purposes, even before the colonization of the Americas and the subsequent slave trade that forcibly removed Africans from their homelands. African women held knowledge of how to identify, harvest, and use many medicinal plants, like cotton-root bark, which was historically used as an abortifacient and contraceptive likely dating back hundreds if not thousands of years. Cotton is in the mallow family along with okra and marshmallow root. Plants in this family have a mucilaginous feature that holds in moisture, and traditionally these plants were used to treat snakebites and dysentery. If harvesting cotton for its root, it is best to do so when it is not flowering or in seed. Instead, wait until the energy is moving into the root system during the fall when the root will have maximum potency.

Eastern Red Cedar

Parts used: *bark, leaves, wood*

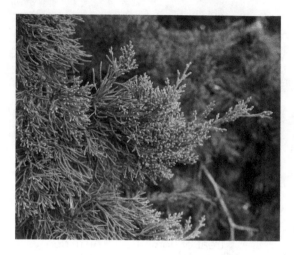

A member of the juniper species but also referred to as eastern cedar, this tree is native to the eastern part of the North American continent. I believe the confusing differences in eastern and western cedar trees give us an example of the myriad different traditions and cultural uses of plants within the sphere of Native American culture. Although there are similarities in the way the two trees are used, there are also vast differences in the way they look, grow, and have been spiritually intertwined into tribes. Just as Indigenous peoples of North America may all be called "Native Americans" and have likenesses, they're also vastly unique from one another. So, when teaching about eastern red cedar, I like to specify how it was used by eastern tribes rather than western tribes.

The Rappahannock Tribe of Virginia created infusions of the juniper berries along with wild ginger to help with asthma. *Juniperus virginiana* is high in vitamin C and was used as a treatment for scurvy by the Haudenosaunee and the Wabanaki. In the 1500s, they shared this "anedda" (a tea) with the French explorer Jacques Cartier, and it is believed this is when it received the nickname "tree of life." The Ojibwe word for the eastern cedar is *giizhikaatag*, and it was used in the formation of canoes along with birch bark. The Cherokee believed eastern cedar to be very sacred and burned its wood only during a ceremony to remove evil spirits. Cedar was also used in the form of smoke medicine, meaning the twigs were burned and the smoke was inhaled while the patient was in an enclosed space. This was done for head colds by the Dakota, Omaha, Pawnee, and Ponca Tribes.

Echinacea

Parts used: *leaves, flowers, roots*

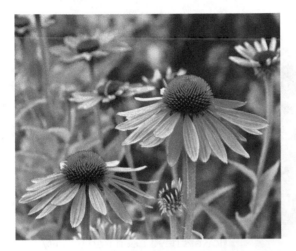

Echinacea grows natively in the middle swath of the country and can be found in pockets on the eastern coast. Also called purple coneflower, the thin, narrow petals range from pink to purple and circle a large, spiny seed cone. Echinacea grows to a height of two to four feet and has narrow, ovate-shaped, and toothed leaves. The tops of the leaves are dark green, and the bottoms have tiny white hairs. Echinacea flowers bloom from June to July and can be foraged from dry, open woods and prairies. The entire plant, including the root, can be harvested and dried for later use or tinctured to extract its potent immune-supporting constituents.

Indigenous tribes considered echinacea a spiritual plant and physical heal-all. Echinacea was one of the more than forty plants the Navajo believed to be "life medicines." The root could be found in medicine pouches and chewed during the Sun Dance ceremony to increase saliva. The root was also chewed to relieve toothaches and decocted to create a wash for treating lice, snakebites, burns, and the eyes. Evidence shows that echinacea supports the respiratory system and strengthens immunity; the two most effective species being *Echinacea purpurea* and *Echinacea angustifolia*. All parts of the plant are medicinal, but among herbalists, the root of echinacea must be included for highest potency. Harvesting the root is best done when the plant is at least three years of age; this is a good reason to take notes on your wildcrafting trips to record areas you have seen plants from year to year. Roots are harvested in the fall by digging twelve inches around the base of the plant until you can pull up the root ball.

Elderberry Tree

Parts used: *flowers, berries*

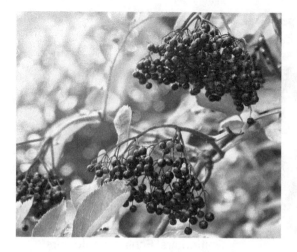

A woody shrub that grows along stream banks and in moist woodlands, elderberry trees can grow twenty to thirty feet tall and can be identified by leaves that are oval-shaped, saw-toothed, and arranged alternately. In late spring, tiny, creamy-white, five-petaled flowers that bloom in large clusters allow for easier identification. When removed fully from their stems, these elderflowers have been traditionally consumed as a tea to quell inflammation and pain and for diuretic, laxative, and perspiration-inducing or fever-breaking purposes. The Mohegan people used this remedy to reduce infantile colic. Native tribes infused water with elderflowers to create what we currently call a hydrosol to use topically for the astringent effects. The Cherokee were known to create external preparations such as soaks, poultices, and salves with the roots and leaves to aid in inflammation and swelling.

The fruit is a small, juicy, slightly sweet, and deep purple berry that forms between July and September. As a precaution, make sure they are fully ripe before harvesting and fully cooked before consuming to avoid digestive discomfort. Dried berries are also widely available at health-food stores and online. Elderberry syrup has become a mainstream way to engage the antiviral, immune-supporting, cough-suppressing, and bronchial and upper-respiratory benefits of this herb and is reminiscent of the way Native peoples have historically used elderberries. Besides using elderberries medicinally, Native Americans also used them to create a natural dye and used the tree's wood in basketry and to fashion bows and arrows, whistles, flutes, and a traditional instrument among Californian tribes called a clapper stick.

Fireweed

Parts used: *leaves, stems, flowers, seeds*

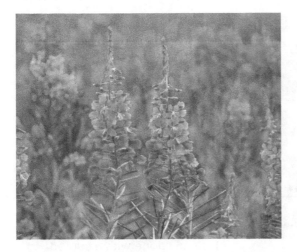

Fireweed is one of the first plants to adopt a home in the soil after a forest fire and is found throughout the Northern Hemisphere. With bright magenta flowers, fireweed can be spotted in sunny meadows and forests, preferring rocky, well-drained soil, and grows up to seven feet tall. The flowers each have four petals and grow in a spike shape, blooming low on the stem. The leaves are narrow and up to four inches long, with smooth sides and a distinctive pale green vein down the middle. Fireweed can be harvested throughout each stage of growth; the young leaves and shoots are a source of vitamin C and were eaten raw by Native Americans. To harvest after blooming, it is best to start pinching the lower leaves off about three to four inches from the base of the flowers and allow the plant to go to seed.

A single fireweed plant produces eighty-thousand seeds, which form as a tuft of silky hairs at the end; this cluster of fluff was used by Native Americans in weaving and as padding. Salish peoples wove fireweed with the down of mountain-goat wool to make blankets. The stems of fireweed were peeled, dried, and twisted for use in fishing nets. The stem pith was used to thicken stews, soups, and poultices. Fireweed tea was consumed to treat stomach and intestinal pain and could be used internally or externally for fungus-related issues such as candida and yeast infections. Eastern tribes used fireweed to treat asthma, whooping cough, and hiccups.

Goldenrod

Parts used: *leaves, flowers*

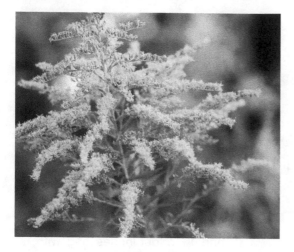

Goldenrod is a tall, herbaceous perennial that blooms prolifically in the late summer. An easy plant to spy, goldenrod grows up to four feet tall in wooded areas and in sunny and dry, open fields. The leaves are narrow and smooth and are two to five inches long. The flowers are small and golden, growing in oblong clusters on the upper end of the branches. Harvesting goldenrod is most efficiently done with a curved harvesting knife by cleanly cutting about four inches below the clusters of flowers. Once harvested, the anise-flavored leaves and flowers can be dried or used fresh in teas or infused into oil for external use. A salve of goldenrod alone or blended with other healing herbs like calendula and yarrow is a helpful item to include in your first aid kit.

Native Americans on both coasts and in between have historically used goldenrod externally as a poultice to treat beestings, open wounds, burns, and a variety of skin conditions. It has also been used to reduce swelling and muscle pain. The roots were used to treat boils and chewed to relieve tooth pain. Internally, goldenrod can be used for bladder, gallbladder, kidney, and digestive disorders; to reduce fever; and to treat gynecological concerns. Due to its antibacterial properties, goldenrod has also been used by traditional healers for sore throats, toothaches, and other oral maladies. Several tribes also considered goldenrod safe for children, using it in cases of fever or excessive crying.

Goldthread Root

Parts used: *roots, stems, leaves*

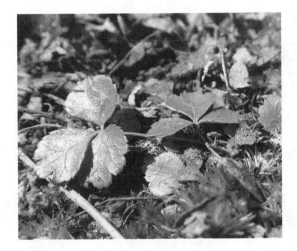

Also called mouthroot or canker-root, one can imagine what this medicinal plant is beneficial for: mouth sores, canker sores, and sores in the throat. Goldthread can also be used for teething babies, thrush, and toothaches. Goldthread root received its name from the appearance of the roots, which are multiple, thin, and threadlike, and golden in hue from the alkaloid present in them known as berberine. Also found in barberry, goldenseal, and turmeric, berberine is a potent antioxidant and anti-inflammatory. According to Mary Siisip Geniusz, a Cree descendant and teacher of Native American ethnobotany, chewing on a piece of the root to quell the pain of an abscessed tooth is more effective than clove oil, which can be used to quell toothaches. Her traditional Indigenous teachings also state that a decoction of this root can expel congestion so quickly that it is not safe to administer to children, because they may choke on the mucus plug. Additionally, goldthread root is classified as a bitter and can be used in your remedies to fill that need, especially when congestion is present in the body.

Goldthread's scientific name is *Coptis trifolia*. The genus *Coptis* includes plants that come from the Ranunculaceae or "little frog" family, and "trifolia" means "three leaved." This plant is small and can be found low to the ground, and it is identified by three scalloped leaflets. When in bloom, you'll find small, solitary white flowers on singular, long, slender, and leafless stems. Goldthread grows throughout the Appalachians in the northeastern part of the United States, most of Canada, and as far south as Alabama.

Horsemint

Parts used: *aerial parts*

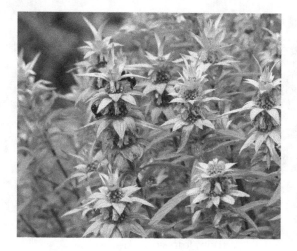

Horsemint is a member of the *Monarda* genus, which encompasses species that may also be called bee balm, Oswego, or wild bergamot. When the term "horse" is added to an herb name, it is a reference to the size of the plant. *Monarda fistulosa* is an unusually tall mint with big, showy, purple or deep red flowers that sit on a bract and are loved by all pollinators, especially hummingbirds, making this an incredibly attractive medicinal plant for your butterfly garden. *Monarda punctata* is a slightly distinct species and sometimes called "spotted horsemint," and the flowers, also on a bract, are a pale purple, but both species are stunning. Like other mints, the stems are square, and the leaves are lance-shaped and toothed and range from one to three inches long.

The healers of southeastern tribes recognized *Monarda punctata* as a stimulant and used it to excite perspiration, increase menstrual flow, and treat obstructions in the reproductive system. They also used it as a diuretic to treat urinary disorders. One traditional Anishinaabe healer by the name of Keewaydinoquay described Oswego tea using the species *Monarda fistulosa* as "the baby-saver tea" because of its ability to calm infantile colic. This remedy can also be used by adults suffering from headaches, toothaches, gingivitis, or insomnia. Horsemint also soothes the digestive tract, helping relieve flatulence, indigestion, bloating, and nausea. The flavor of *Monarda fistulosa* is like that of bergamot, the citrus fruit that is used to flavor Earl Grey tea, so blending this herb with a tea is a pleasant way of consuming it.

Huckleberry

Parts used: *berries, leaves, stems, flowers*

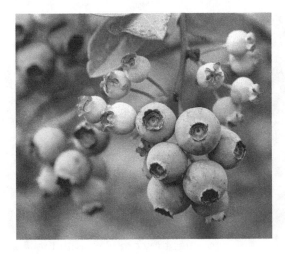

There are several species of huckleberry shrubs growing throughout the North American continent. They have thin branches and broad, flat leaves with a pointed tip. In the spring, they bloom small white to pink flowers. The berries are a quarter inch in diameter and come in a wide variety of colors, from red to dark purple.

Huckleberries were not only part of Indigenous peoples' diets and medicines, but the harvest season was also a time to connect with family and friends from seasons past and to celebrate and recharge before fall fishing and winterizing their villages. These harvests brought together tribes from different linguistic groups, which is why they are also considered to have a spiritual and cultural significance. Henry David Thoreau believed the first known documentation of this berry occurred in 1615 by explorer Samuel de Champlain, who noticed the Algonquin people collecting and drying a small berry that he called "blue" for winter use. It is noted that in addition to huckleberries being a food, they were also "comfit for the sick." Native Americans would create fire-driven driers or smokers to preserve the berries, sometimes smashing them into cakes and wrapping them with leaves or bark for storage. Additionally, tribes exchanged these dried huckleberries as currency with European settlers.

The leaves, stems, and flowers were infused to create a tea and also used to purify the blood, to induce labor, and as a diuretic. The Cheyenne made a decoction of the bark for colds, and an infusion of the fruit and leaves was given to mothers after childbirth to help them regain strength. The Nez Percé, Chinook, and other Northwest tribes thought of huckleberry as a heart medicine and ceremonial food. Huckleberries do in fact have heart-healthy antioxidants and anthocyanins, immune-supportive and scurvy-preventing vitamin C, and skin-protecting vitamin A. Last, huckleberries are a source of potassium, which supports healthy water balance and supports the kidneys and bladder.

Lousewort

Parts used: *flowers, leaves, roots*

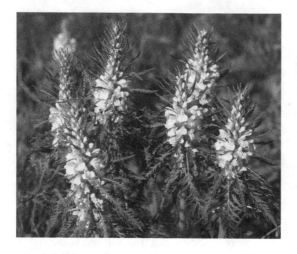

In herbalism today, lousewort is commonly referred to as wood betony and is a popular medicinal plant in the mint family. Growing low to the ground, lousewort grows from five to fourteen inches high and has the appearance of fine hairs; the body of the plant includes up to five erect, unbranched stems that grow in a clump. The leaves are three to five inches in length and form a crown as they grow up, with the inside leaves being smaller. The aerial parts of the plant can be harvested when the flowers bloom in mid- to late summer; the flowers grow erect and are tubular and yellow or purple. Aerial parts harvested can be dried and stored for later use. Lousewort can be found in cleared lots, moist, open woods, and in thickets throughout most of North America.

Many tribes used lousewort for digestive discomforts such as diarrhea and stomachaches, including those induced by menstruation. The Haudenosaunee also considered it a heart medicine, creating infusions with the root, whereas the Chippewa used the roots for anemia and in steam baths to soothe the legs and knees. The Menominee Tribe believed the root could enhance love when carried by the courter, or the root was cooked and consumed to regain a loved one's admiration. Physically, the Native Americans believed this herb to have an aphrodisiac effect. Today, herbalists recommend wood betony as a sedative, reducing stress, anxiety, and the muscle tension that comes along with those feelings.

Passionflower

Parts used: *leaves, vine, flowers, roots*

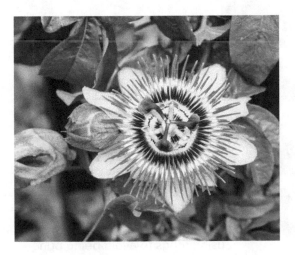

Passionflower's name may have been inspired by the passion of Christ, and its flowers were used as a visual aid of Christ's crucifixion by missionaries attempting to convert Indigenous peoples.

The flowers are saucer-shaped and pale to dark purple, and they bloom from June to September; they're unique and highly recognizable. An aggressive growing vine, passionflower can grow more than eight feet long and spread three to six feet wide. If the plant doesn't have a structure to climb, it will just weave itself throughout the landscape, potentially suffocating other plants. The leaves stem directly from the vine, have three to five lobes, and taper to sharp points. Tendrils support the plant in trellising. In late summer, it produces egg-shaped fruit two inches in size that are called "maypops" in the south due to the way they pop when stepped on.

The first reported use of passionflower was by the Aztecs, who consumed the tea to induce rest. The Algonquin-speaking tribes reportedly used it to "inspire tranquility." Traditional healers also recognized passionflower's ability to quell pain, especially in the case of dysmenorrhea (menstrual cramps). Some Native American tribes spread poultices created from the root of passionflower on inflamed areas to draw out inflammation. They would also give the juice of the root to weaning babies or drop the juice into ears for pain and infection. Roots are rarely employed today; instead, the leaves and flowers are made into medicines for stress, anxiety, irritability, sleeplessness, and postpartum depression.

Prickly Pear

Parts used: *body, fruit*

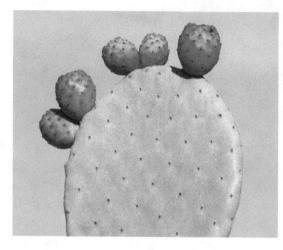

Prickly pear is an edible cactus found in the southwestern part of the United States and down through Mexico, growing in large clumps. They are also called "nopales" or "paddle cactus" because of the broad and flat shape of their body. Prickly pears have round nodes that protrude out from their body, bloom from May to July, and can be harvested in August. Harvesting can be done using tongs to avoid being punctured by the glochids (spines). It is also best to use gloves and cover exposed skin. Grasp the nodule firmly with the tongs and twist or snap it off at the base where it connects to the plant. Before consuming, the glochids can be removed by scrubbing with a vegetable brush with gloved hands.

Native Americans used the innards of prickly pear as a burn dressing and for other inflammations of the skin. The Lakota considered it a snakebite remedy, and the Shoshoni and the Pawnee applied the inner pulp to cuts and wounds to aid with the pain. The Pima Tribe of Arizona heated the plant and applied it to the breasts as a galactagogue, a substance that increases breast-milk flow. The young round body of the cactus was cut into strips, boiled, and eaten; the fruits were mashed into jelly, juice, or syrup. The Apache mashed the fruit of the species *Opuntia leptocaulis* and drank it as a narcotic, and the Flathead Tribe considered prickly pear an analgesic, applying it for backaches.

Sagebrush

Parts used: *leaves, stems*

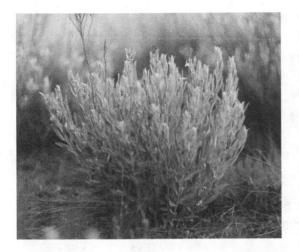

Growing in the western part of North America, sagebrush is a gnarly looking woody shrub that prefers full sun and dry, rocky soils. Sagebrush shrubs grow two to nine feet tall, and their leaves are a silvery blue gray, with three lobes on the end of each leaf. Sagebrush is aromatic and smells distinctly of camphor. It flowers in the fall. The Paiute people used sagebrush in the building of shelters and would even fashion this shrub into snowshoes and other articles of clothing. Ceremonial sagebrush was patted on dancers to make them spiritually clean, used in the creation of the sweat-lodge frame, and burned during ceremonies to kill airborne illnesses.

A tea made of sagebrush was widely used by many western tribes as a respiratory aid, cold remedy, cough medicine, and as a diaphoretic or sweat-inducing plant. The stems and leaves were decocted to create a throat syrup, and the leaves were put in the nose to stop it from running. An herbal steam was also inhaled in cases of head and chest colds, or a poultice would be created to put on the chest of the ill. Many western tribes used sagebrush for digestive disorders and as an antidiarrheal. The Navajo consumed sagebrush tea to relieve headaches and for postpartum pain, and newborn babies were bathed in warm antiseptic baths of sagebrush. Sagebrush could also be used as a wash for sores and pimples and to ease muscle pain and athlete's foot.

Stinging Nettle

Parts used: *leaves, stems, roots*

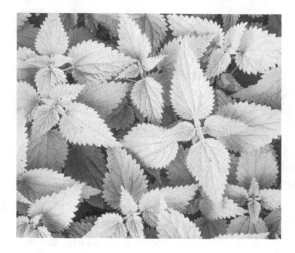

There are several species of stinging nettle, or *Urtica*; some were introduced to the North American continent, whereas others are native, and one or more species grows throughout the continent. They all share the trait of having stinging hairs (nettles) that, when touched, will irritate the skin. Stinging nettle plants grow from three to six feet tall. The leaves are heart-shaped, serrated, and a deep green, and the stem is hollow to solid, fibrous, and tough. Nettle flowers in late spring through late autumn, and the flowers aren't very exciting in color; they are small and reddish brown or greenish white. Nettle plants can be found growing in moist and shady spaces but spread easily past those zones through their rhizomes. To harvest, be prepared by wearing long sleeves and gloves, and place the plant in a paper bag or box after cutting it with a pair of pliers. Hang upside down to dry, and once dried, the nettles will not sting any longer.

The Cherokee and the Lakota used nettles to treat digestive issues, and other eastern tribes recognized it for its ability to heal conditions of the urinary tract. The Cree used nettle decoctions to "keep blood flowing after childbirth," which is likely a reference to the iron content we now know nettle leaves to have. The Abenaki Tribe knew California nettle to be a styptic, meaning it can stop bleeding, and they used powdered leaves as a snuff to stop nosebleeds. This external use of nettle was common among tribes to treat wounds. Patients with arthritis and rheumatic conditions were also patted with fresh nettles or washed with the decocted root to ease inflammation and pain.

Sumac

Parts used: *berries, bark*

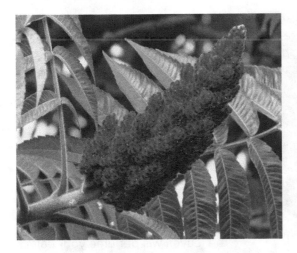

Sumac can be a tall shrub or a tree that grows from twenty-four to thirty feet around streams or swamps, at the edges of wooded areas, and along roadsides or railways. To identify a sumac tree, start by inspecting the leaves, flowers, and berries. The leaves start as a shiny green and will evolve their color from gold to red in the fall; they are fernlike and oblong-shaped and grow sixteen to twenty-four inches long. The flowers grow in a cone shape before becoming berries that form dense cone-shaped clusters that will begin to droop from their weight. The berries are small and have a fuzzy texture, and in the fall, they are bright red and gradually become a deeper red in the winter. Late summer is the best time to harvest sumac berries. Look for clusters that are bright red; when touched, they will feel slightly sticky and taste tart.

Eastern tribes used sumac to treat bladder discomfort and kidney issues, including urinary tract infections. The Cherokee created sumac-berry infusions or bark decoctions to soak the skin when sunburned and blistered. The Chippewa used the blossoms to make a mouthwash for teething babies and used the roots as a cold remedy. The berries are high in vitamin C and antioxidants, making them ideal to prevent colds and speed the healing process. Sumac was also used by multiple tribes for women's health: before childbirth to ease the pain and in cases of hemorrhaging after childbirth.

Western Cedar Tree

Parts used: *leaves*

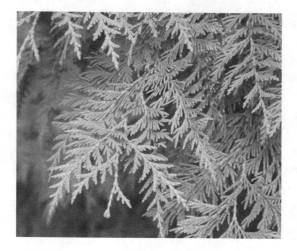

Western cedar is a tree common throughout the Pacific Northwest; these trees can live for more than 1,000 years and grow more than 150 feet tall. The western cedar is not actually a true cedar; its scientific name is *Thuja plicata*, and it belongs to the cypress family. The foliage of these trees is distinct and quite beautiful: It is short, flat, and soft, and is fernlike in appearance. When pressed in your hands, the leaves will perfume your palm with the terpene thujone. Terpenes are scent-emitting chemicals of the plant. Due to this aromatic oil, which is a natural disinfectant, cedar has been traditionally used to fumigate a space in cases of contagious diseases such as smallpox.

In Salish, the names for this tree translate to "long-life giver" and "mother" because western red cedar trees were able to provide for these tribes from life to death. The medicine within the leaf has antimicrobial and antifungal properties. The leaves can be made into a salve or tincture or consumed as a tea. When ingested, cedar improves immune function by stimulating white blood cells. You can also bring this medicinal plant to a simmer in a pot of water, remove it from the heat, and place your head while covered with a towel over the steam to inhale the sinus-clearing and cough-reducing benefits. To take advantage of cedar's antifungal properties, the tincture or an infused oil can be applied topically. In the case of foot fungus, simply soak feet in a bath of warm water infused with cedar leaves.

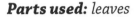

Yaupon Holly

Parts used: *leaves*

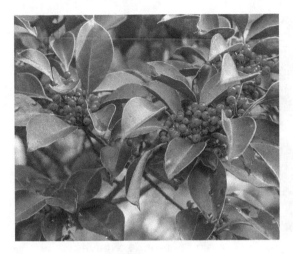

An evergreen shrub, yaupon holly can be found in the eastern part of the United States in open fields and swamps, growing up to twenty-four feet tall. The leaves grow in a chaotic pattern up to one inch in length and are an ovate shape, bright green, and spaced out one-half to one inch apart. This species is called *Ilex vomitoria* due to the nausea the red berries that appear in the fall can induce. You can harvest the leaves by cutting off a tree limb and hanging it to dry or by drying single leaves.

The Native Americans made a "black drink" with yaupon leaves that they called "Osceola," which was the name of a god recognized by the Creek people and later the name of a Seminole leader. The Seminoles also used yaupon tea to reduce instances of nightmares, sleepwalking, and sleep talking. The leaves were so revered that Native Americans traveled to consume and trade this tea sometimes as far as Mexico, where they exchanged it for cacao and blended the two together to drink. In the book *Travels of William Bartram* (1791), Bartram wrote, "Our Chief with the rest of the white people in town, took their seats according to order: tobacco and pipes were brought; the calumet was lighted and smoked, circulating to the usual forms and ceremony; and afterward, black drink con-clude the feast." A natural stimulant and high in antioxidants, yaupon tea inspired connection, increased endurance, and protected the immune systems of the Native Americans.

Yerba Santa

Parts used: *leaves, stems*

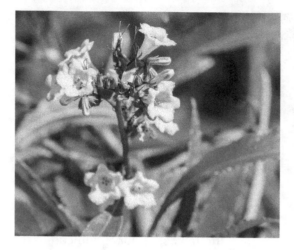

Yerba santa is a shrub that grows up to ten feet tall with a width average of three feet. Growing only in a few western states, including Arizona, Nevada, and New Mexico, yerba santa prefers rocky slopes and ridges and thrives in places disturbed by fire or construction. The leaves of yerba santa have a tough leathery feel and, when mature, will be sticky to the touch due to their resin content. The leaves grow three to four inches long and alternate along the stem. The flowers bloom from July to August and are white and purple in color; they are small and arranged in clusters of six to ten flowers.

"Yerba santa" translates to "holy weed" or "holy grass" and has traditionally been revered for its ability to heal respiratory illnesses. The Shoshone and the Paiute Tribes created decoctions with the leaves and stems to use as an expectorant, expelling mucus from the lungs, lessening cough, and even treating whooping cough and tuberculosis. The leaves were also chewed or smoked as a pulmonary aid. Many Native Americans believe that the land will supply the right medicine for their needs. For example, yerba santa can be used to fight the respiratory effects of wildfires that occur in the western states that the plant grows in. It has also gained the name "fire follower" because it will readily seed or spread by rhizome after a fire. Yerba santa can reduce inflammation of the lungs, throat, and sinuses, so consuming it as a tea or tincture after fire exposure may reduce respiratory damage.

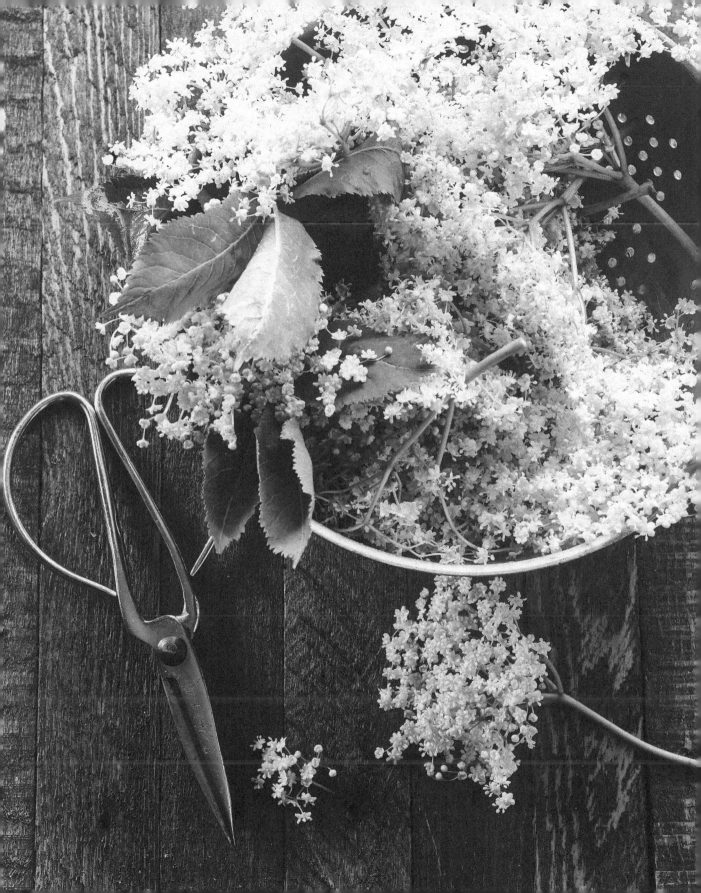

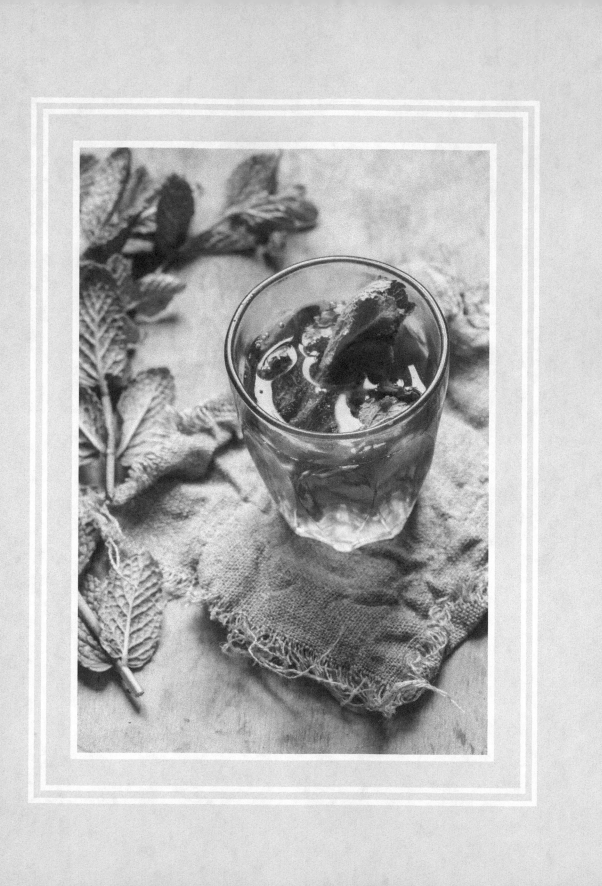

PART III

Native American Remedies for Health and Wellness

In this section, seventy-five unique remedies are offered to educate you further on the plants that were traditionally used by Native Americans, as well as waking up your creativity in your herbal apothecary. The remedies vary in complexity and the quantity of herbs used. Many of the remedies are rounded out by herbs that are found in other cultures but have their foundation in Indigenous wisdom. In herbalism, it is not uncommon for one herb to support a variety of body systems in different ways, so it is always an adventure to learn more about a medicinal plant and how a remedy created with it will do more than quiet a cough or lessen a headache. This section is arranged by ailment, including such common ailments as anxiety, immunity problems, hormone issues, and skin conditions. Although a remedy may be listed under a particular ailment, it is worthwhile to read through all the remedies and recognize the ones that can be used daily to ward off illness and support your general health daily. Doing so is especially worthwhile in the energy and nutrition sections, because both offer remedies that are nutritious substitutes to conventional foods. As you learn more about the uses of herbs, you'll discover how to make substitutions in these remedies based on the plants you have access to and become familiar with.

Diarrhea-Relief Tea

Makes 2 cups   **PREP TIME:** *10 minutes*

Blackberry leaves and roots were used by several Native American tribes in cases of diarrhea and even dysentery. The astringency of the tannins found in the root and leaves of the blackberry plant constricts mucus membranes in the intestinal tract, effectively reducing the frequency of bowel movements and supporting the return of firmer stools.

Chamomile reduces inflammation around the gut lining and the stress and anxiety that could be contributing to excessive movement of the bowels. Peppermint leaves balance this tea formulation by relaxing the bowels, lessening cramps, calming the smooth muscles of the intestinal tract, and increasing coolness within the digestive system. Ginger is another digestive herb that quells nausea and is antibacterial and antiviral, so it may help ward off the bad bugs that cause diarrhea.

INGREDIENTS

**1 cup dried
blackberry root**
**½ cup dried
chamomile flowers**
**½ cup dried
peppermint leaves**
**Sprinkle of
dried gingerroot**
**8 to 12 ounces
boiling water**

SUPPLIES

Large mixing bowl
**Gloves, for blending
(optional)**
Storage container

INSTRUCTIONS

1. To make the tea blend, in a large bowl, combine the blackberry root, chamomile, peppermint, and gingerroot. Stir well to combine. Transfer to a clean, airtight container.

2. When ready to consume, put 2 teaspoons of the tea blend in a fillable, reusable, or disposable tea bag, or stainless steel tea infuser. Cover with the boiling water, and let steep for 10 to 20 minutes before consuming.

Goldthread and Turmeric Electuary

Makes 1 cup   **PREP TIME:** *30 minutes*

An electuary is a synergistic blend of raw honey and powdered herbs, vegetables, and/or fruit to be consumed for medicinal and health-promoting purposes. Honey is anti-bacterial, anti-inflammatory, and immune-modulating. Combine this sweet nectar with the nutritional and medicinal benefits of plants, and you have a natural catalyst that drives the medicine of your plants deeper into the cells of your body—and it also tastes delicious.

Goldthread and turmeric are both roots containing considerable amounts of berberine, a potent compound that offers protection from harmful organisms, boosts the immune system, calms inflammation, and heals tissue. This electuary can also be used topically on sores inside and outside of the mouth and added to warm water to create a mouthwash. Both roots in this formula contain compounds that are lipophilic (lipid-loving), meaning they're attracted to fats; for this reason, coconut oil is incorporated into this electuary recipe.

INGREDIENTS

1 tablespoon
  ground turmeric
1 teaspoon
  goldthread powder
½ teaspoon ground
  cinnamon (optional)
¾ cup honey
1 tablespoon coconut oil

SUPPLIES

Small bowl
Mixing spatula
Large bowl
Sanitized storage
  container

INSTRUCTIONS

1. In a small bowl, combine the turmeric, goldthread, and cinnamon (if using).

2. In a separate large bowl, combine the honey and coconut oil. Stir to blend well.

3. Slowly begin to blend the powdered herbs into the honey–coconut oil mixture, ensuring all herbs get coated with honey. Once fully blended, transfer to a clean, airtight container, and store in the refrigerator for up to 6 months.

Herbal-Infused Oil for Pain

Makes 1 cup   **PREP TIME:** *20 minutes, plus 2 weeks to infuse*

Named after a prophet, Saint-John's-wort is a medicinal plant native to the eastern part of North America. The word "wort" is an Old English word meaning plant, root, or herb and is often used in relation to a plant having specific affinities for an organ system, e.g., "liverwort" or "lungwort." Traditionally, preparations of Saint-John's-wort have been used for psychological support, to help with seasonal depression, and to help ease physical pain like sciatica or nerve pain. Combined with arnica, this infused oil can be used for bruises and joint pain. The pain-relieving terpenes of hops are especially helpful for sore, tense, spasmodic muscles. If you choose to include cayenne, it can suppress the neurotransmitter that signals pain to the brain; however, it will add extra warmth and should be applied with gloves if hands cannot be washed adequately.

INGREDIENTS

¼ **cup dried Saint-John's-wort**
¼ **cup dried arnica flowers**
2 tablespoons dried hops
1 tablespoon cayenne (optional)
1 to 2 cups carrier oil

SUPPLIES

2-cup widemouthed glass jar, sanitized
Cheesecloth and metal sieve
Sanitized storage container

INSTRUCTIONS

1. In a 2-cup widemouthed glass jar, combine the Saint-John's-wort, arnica, hops, and cayenne (if using).

2. Add the oil, covering the herbs completely. Close the jar, and shake. Add more oil if the herbs are not covered completely. Place by a sunny window, and shake periodically.

3. After 2 weeks, using a metal sieve and/or cheese-cloth, strain the herbs from the oil. Store in a clean, airtight container away from light. For optimum freshness, it's best to use this oil within 6 months.

Jamaican Dogwood Tea

Makes 1 cup   **PREP TIME:** *20 minutes*

Jamaican dogwood is a tree native to Florida, the Caribbean, and Central America. It is also referred to as the Florida fish fuddle tree, due to the Taino people's observations that extracts from the tree could sedate fish. In fact, one of its herbal benefits is nerve sedation as well as nervous excitability. Jamaican dogwood is well-known in herbalism for its ability to quell pain quickly. The bark of this tree is used to treat anxiety, headaches, nerve pain, and sleeplessness. Its ability to lessen spasms makes it useful for back pain as well as menstrual pain. Jamaican dogwood is best for acute cases of pain and insomnia and is not ideal for long-term use.

Cinnamon increases circulation, moving the blood throughout the body, breaking up stagnation and calming inflammation on its own, but it also helps mask the bitter flavor of the Jamaican dogwood. However, if you are still unable to tolerate the flavor of this tea, you can create a Jamaican dogwood tincture by referring to the Cotton-Root Bark Tincture (page 120) recipe.

INGREDIENTS

8 ounces water
1 teaspoon dried Jamaican dogwood bark
1 teaspoon ground cinnamon
Honey or sugar, for serving

SUPPLIES

Small saucepan
Strainer

INSTRUCTIONS

1. In a small saucepan, combine the water, dogwood bark, and cinnamon. Bring to a boil over medium heat, about 10 to 15 minutes. Remove from the heat. Let steep for an hour (if possible).

2. Strain the mixture into a mug, and add honey to taste.

Fresh Wild Lettuce Tincture

Makes 1 cup   **PREP TIME:** *1 hour, plus at least 1 week to infuse*

The scientific name of wild lettuce is *Lactuca canadensis,* "lac" is derived from the Greek word for milk and "canadensis" for the first known land it was found on, Canada. Wild lettuce is an invasive weed that grows almost entirely throughout North America. The leaves of wild lettuce are serrated and resemble dandelion leaves, and the stalk is like a thistle stalk and can grow up to five feet tall. Also referred to as lettuce opium, this plant doesn't contain opium, but it does contain pain-relieving and sedating compounds called lactucarium. If you break the stalk of wild lettuce, a latex will ooze out. It's in this sap that the medicinal benefits are found, making a fresh herb preparation more beneficial than a dried herb. The milky juice of wild lettuce can also soothe the symptoms caused by contact with poison ivy.

INGREDIENTS

1 cup fresh wild
   lettuce leaves and
   stalks, chopped
1½ cups grain alcohol

SUPPLIES

Cutting board and knife
Glass jar
Blender (optional)
Metal sieve
   and/or cheesecloth
Storage container

INSTRUCTIONS

1. Put the chopped lettuce in a jar.

2. Add enough alcohol to cover the lettuce.

3. Let the alcohol-and-plant infusion sit for 4 weeks, shaking the jar regularly.
   Optional: For maximum extraction of the compound lactucarium, you can place the alcohol-plant mixture in a blender on low speed for 10 to 15 seconds to break down plant matter further. This mixture will be ready to strain in a week.

4. Using a sieve and/or cheesecloth, strain the mixture into a new container.

Allergy Tea with Goldenrod

Makes ¾ cup   **PREP TIME:** *10 minutes*

Goldenrod wrongfully gets accused of causing hay fever and seasonal allergies. Its pollen doesn't circulate through the air like that of wind-pollinated plants such as ragweed, whose growth coincides with goldenrod's and is one of the main culprits of the seasonal allergies suffered by millions in the late summer. Indigenous peoples believe that the medicine we need at any given time makes itself present at the time we are in the most need, and goldenrod is an example of this belief. Goldenrod grows abundantly just in time to relieve seasonal allergy symptoms.

This tea blend contains goldenrod and rooibos, which are powerful sources of the bioflavonoids quercetin and rutin. Quercetin and rutin reduce inflammation and effectively block histamine, the chemical that incites the symptoms associated with allergies. The astringency of goldenrod and nettles in this formula supports the bronchial passages, and nettles also contribute allergy-fighting B and C vitamins. Elderflower is a source of chlorogenic acids, compounds that have been shown to decrease sensitivity to common allergens. The blend of these powerful herbs is best consumed before allergy symptoms show up.

INGREDIENTS

½ cup rooibos leaves

½ cup dried goldenrod

¼ cup dried elderflower

¼ cup dried
  nettle leaves

8 to 12 ounces
  boiling water

SUPPLIES

Large mixing bowl

Gloves, for blending
  (optional)

Storage container

INSTRUCTIONS

1. To make the tea blend, in a large bowl, combine the rooibos, goldenrod, elderflower, and nettle leaves. Stir well to blend. Transfer to a clean, airtight container. Dried herbal teas retain potency for up to 1 year if stored correctly.

2. To make a cup of tea, steep 2 teaspoons of the herbal tea blend in the boiling water for 5 to 10 minutes.

Passionflower Stress-Relief Tea

Makes 1 cup   **PREP TIME:** *10 minutes*

Passionflower roots, leaves, and flowers were used in multiple ways by Native Americans, but today only the aerial parts of this medicinal plant are commonly used to relieve stress and anxiety. They are also used as a sedative and pain reliever. Passionflower can be a great soother when the mind is working overtime, and in this tea blend, skullcap is added to help stop circular thoughts. Skullcap creates a headband effect around the skull, inducing a heaviness that is welcome when you've become restless. Peppermint is the base of this stress-relieving tea and can provide digestive support to a nervous tummy and bring about peacefulness. A touch of lavender is added for its ability to induce a sense of calm and serenity. This tea can be consumed at any time of day, but keep in mind that it may carry you into a slumber, so be prepared to nap after sipping.

INGREDIENTS

½ cup dried
   peppermint leaves
¼ cup dried
   passionflower
2 tablespoons
   dried skullcap
1 to 2 tablespoons
   dried lavender
8 to 12 ounces
   boiling water

SUPPLIES

Large mixing bowl
Gloves, for blending
   (optional)
Storage container

INSTRUCTIONS

1. To make the tea blend, in a large bowl, combine the peppermint, passionflower, skullcap, and lavender. Stir to blend well. Transfer to a clean, airtight container. Dried herbal teas retain potency for up to 1 year if stored correctly.

2. To make a cup of tea, steep 2 teaspoons of the herbal tea blend in the boiling water for 5 to 10 minutes.

Skullcap Nerve-Support Tea

Makes 1 cup   **PREP TIME:** *10 minutes*

Skullcap is a medicinal herb that grows in several pockets of North America. The Miwok people of Northern California used narrow-leaf skullcap to wash sore eyes. The species referred to as hairy and hoary skullcap grows primarily in eastern states and was used by the Cherokee to treat diarrhea and breast pain, to speed the expulsion of afterbirth, and as a kidney medicine. The Delaware Tribe used marsh skullcap for laxative benefits, and the Ojibwe considered it a heart medicine. Blue skullcap, or *Scutellaria lateriflora*, is the species that grows most widely across the continent and is the most common you'll find in dried-herb form through retailers. This species is used in the same ways as other species and was also used by the Haudenosaunee as a throat aid.

In modern herbalism, skullcap is categorized as an herbal nervine, soothing the nervous system, inducing sleep through a heaviness of the head. Passionflower is another sedating nervine that lessens stress and anxiety and is written about in detail on page 51.

INGREDIENTS

½ **cup dried spearmint**
¼ **cup dried skullcap**
¼ **cup**
  dried passionflower
8 to 12 ounces
  boiling water

SUPPLIES

Medium mixing bowl
Gloves, for blending
  (optional)
Storage container

INSTRUCTIONS

1. To make the tea blend, in a medium mixing bowl, combine the spearmint, skullcap, and passionflower. Stir to blend well. Transfer to a clean, airtight container. Dried herbal teas retain potency for up to 1 year if stored correctly.

2. To make a cup of tea, steep 2 teaspoons of the herbal tea blend in the boiling water for 5 to 10 minutes.

Tension-Release Tea

Makes 1 cup   **PREP TIME:** *10 minutes*

Nervines strengthen the nervous system, further equipping your body to respond to pain. These medicinal plants help ease and soothe pain through toning and nourishing the affected areas, and they also strengthen our ability to cope with stress. Nervines fall into four categories: nerve tonics, nerve sedatives, nervine demulcents, and nerve stimulants. Lousewort, the featured herb in this tea, is also known as wood betony and is a nerve tonic that tonifies the digestive system in rhythm with the nervous system. It also melts tension that develops around our necks and shoulders. Oat straw is a highly nutritious nerve demulcent and is a source of calming B vitamins, magnesium, calcium, and silica. Lemon balm offers a calm focus, and studies have found it improves ADHD symptoms and is safe for children. The sweet licorice-like scent of anise hyssop can ease frazzled nerves and reduce pain. If you're able to grow and harvest this beautiful herb yourself, it can bring joy to your cup of tea.

INGREDIENTS

¼ **cup dried lousewort**

¼ **cup dried oat straw**

¼ **cup dried lemon balm leaves**

¼ **cup dried anise hyssop**

8 to 12 ounces boiling water

SUPPLIES

Medium mixing bowl

Gloves, for blending (optional)

Storage container

INSTRUCTIONS

1. To make the tea blend, in a medium bowl, combine the lousewort, oat straw, lemon balm leaves, and anise hyssop. Stir to blend well. Transfer to a clean, airtight container. Dried herbal teas retain potency for up to 1 year if stored correctly.

2. To make a cup of tea, steep 2 teaspoons of the herbal tea blend in the boiling water for 5 to 10 minutes.

Heart-Strength Tea

Makes 1½ cups   **PREP TIME:** *10 minutes*

This tea is a blend of native and nonnative plants from North America that work together to strengthen the heart. Linden, also known as American basswood, is a native tree growing from North Dakota down to Texas and all the states toward the east coast. Linden flowers are used to support healthy heart circulation and are excellent for nervous-system conditions. Hibiscus, a nonnative, tropical plant, is traditionally used in Africa and the Caribbean. Current research shows tea made with this bright red flower may support the reduction of hypertension. Varied species of hawthorn grow natively throughout North America. The bark, berries, and flowers of this tree are used medicinally, and it is documented that the Cherokee consumed bark infusions as heart medicine. Motherwort was introduced to the Native Americans by settlers and currently grows throughout the entire continent. Motherwort is bitter in flavor and can be used to aid in digestion and calm frazzled nerves.

INGREDIENTS

½ cup dried
  linden flowers
½ cup dried
  hibiscus flowers
¼ cup dried
  hawthorn flowers
¼ cup dried
  motherwort leaves
8 to 12 ounces
  boiling water

SUPPLIES

Medium mixing bowl
Gloves, for blending
  (optional)
Storage container

INSTRUCTIONS

1. To make the tea blend, in a medium bowl, combine the linden, hibiscus, hawthorn, and motherwort. Stir to blend well. Transfer to a clean, airtight container. Dried herbal teas retain potency for up to 1 year if stored correctly.

2. To make a cup of tea, steep 2 teaspoons of the herbal tea blend in the boiling water for 10 to 20 minutes.

Homemade Stevia Extract

Makes ½ cup

PREP TIME: *10 minutes, plus at least 24 hours to infuse* / **COOK TIME:** *20 minutes*

Stevia is a small bush native to Paraguay. Its leaves are two hundred to three hundred times sweeter than sugar but don't contain calories or cause blood-sugar imbalances. The Guarani, the Indigenous people of South America, where several species of stevia grow, have used this plant ceremonially, medicinally, and in food preparation since pre-Hispanic times. Stevia gained popularity in the United States in the late 1900s, and by the early 2000s, stevia-sweetened products were heavily marketed. This amount of commercialization of one plant has led to global overconsumption that negatively affects Indigenous people like the Guarani, who have historically used the plant and carry the traditional knowledge of its usage. One simple step you can take to fight against the commercialization of stevia is to grow your own stevia plants. Since they are not cold-hardy, they can be brought inside and placed under lights during the winter, and even one to two small plants can be enough to satisfy your basic needs.

INGREDIENTS

½ cup fresh stevia
   leaves, chopped
1 cup vodka

SUPPLIES

Cutting board and knife
2-cup glass jar
Metal sieve and/or
   cheesecloth
Small saucepan
Glass storage jar with
   lid or dropper bottles

INSTRUCTIONS

1. Put the chopped stevia leaves in a 2-cup glass jar, and pour in enough vodka to cover. Seal the jar, and shake. Let infuse for 24 to 48 hours.

2. Strain the mixture over a small saucepan. Cook the alcohol off by heating for 20 minutes over low heat; do not boil. Remove from the heat. Let cool to room temperature before storing in a glass jar or dropper bottle for up to 6 months.

Hawthorn-Ginkgo Extract

Makes 1 cup   **PREP TIME:** *30 minutes, plus at least 4 weeks to infuse*

The combination of these two plants supports healthy circulation. The Native Americans have considered hawthorn to be a heart medicine for centuries, and ginkgo biloba has been important in traditional Chinese medicine for thousands of years. The combination of these two circulatory herbs is popular in Europe for treating Alzheimer's disease, headaches, tinnitus, and diabetes. Ginkgo biloba is often associated with the brain, and for good reason: Research has shown that this medicinal plant's antioxidant properties protect the lipids in the brain from oxidative stress. Hawthorn has flavonoids that increase the metabolism in the heart muscles by dilating the peripheral and coronary vessels.

Creating your own herbal products saves money in addition to allowing you to be aware of every ingredient used and of its quality. These are two medicinal herbs that can easily be bought economically by the ounce at your local health-food store or through online vendors.

INGREDIENTS

¼ cup dried
  ginkgo leaves
¼ cup dried
  hawthorn leaves
1½ cups vodka

SUPPLIES

2- to 4-cup glass jar
  with lid
Metal sieve
Storage container
Funnel
Storage bottles

INSTRUCTIONS

1. In a 2- or 4-cup glass jar, combine the ginkgo and hawthorn.

2. Add enough alcohol to cover by 1 inch. Seal the jar tightly, and label.

3. Place the jar in a cool, shady spot, and gently shake every few days for 4 to 6 weeks.

4. To strain, place a sieve over an open container, and pour in the tincture extract. Gently press the plant material to release all fluid.

5. Using a funnel, pour the fluid into dropper bottles. Store for up to 2 years.

Memory Support Tea

Makes 1½ cups   **PREP TIME:** *10 minutes*

In recent years, nootropics have grown in popularity in the herbal-supplement industry. The word "nootropic" is derived from the Greek words "noos" (mind) and "tropic" (toward). This category of herbs and nutrients supports cognitive function—specifically, that of memory, focus, and creativity. It also prevents mental decline due to Alzheimer's disease and dementia.

The first three herbs in this formulation are commonly used in Ayurvedic medicine, the natural system of medicine practiced in India. Studies show that gotu kola stimulates capillaries, helping improve brain function. Research also suggests it may improve the brain's ability to use glucose for energy. Tulsi is an aromatic herb that serves many purposes within the body, including blood-sugar support and the reduction of cortisol levels. The overproduction of cortisol due to stress will lessen our abilities to focus and keep memories. Bacopa promotes memory and focus and may be helpful in the presence of brain trauma. Rosemary is a source of antioxidants and is traditionally used to improve short-term memory. Even just the scent of rosemary before reading can enhance retention.

INGREDIENTS

½ **cup dried gotu kola**
½ **cup dried tulsi**
¼ **cup dried bacopa**
¼ **cup rosemary**
8 to 12 ounces
   boiling water

SUPPLIES

Medium mixing bowl
Gloves, for blending
   (optional)
Storage container

INSTRUCTIONS

1. To make the tea blend, in a medium bowl, combine the gotu kola, tulsi, bacopa, and rosemary. Stir to blend well. Transfer to a clean, airtight container. Dried herbal teas retain potency for up to 1 year if stored correctly.

2. To make a cup of tea, steep 2 teaspoons of the herbal tea blend in the boiling water for 5 to 10 minutes.

Boneset Tea

Makes 1 cup   **PREP TIME:** *10 minutes*

Boneset is prized in herbalism for its ability to restore white-blood-cell count by stimulating the health of the bone marrow. It can alleviate pain from chronic health conditions and help break a fever from a cold or flu by moving fluids through the body and dispersing heat. Boneset opens the elimination pathways of both the kidneys and liver, allowing for toxins to be transported out quickly, making it important to hydrate well while taking boneset.

The flavor of boneset is bitter, and all bitter plants support the liver by increasing gastrointestinal juices to move bile through faster, increasing the speed of assimilation of fats and toxins. Bitter flavors will be less tolerable, making it unlikely you will take in more than needed. This tea also incorporates the antiviral support and milder flavor of lemon balm and the demulcent action of marshmallow root. Drinking this tea upon the onset of symptoms can reduce the length and severity of sickness, soothe irritated mucus membranes, and reduce coughing.

INGREDIENTS

½ cup dried
   lemon balm
¼ cup dried boneset
¼ cup dried
   marshmallow root
8 to 12 ounces
   boiling water

SUPPLIES

Medium mixing bowl
Gloves, for blending
   (optional)

INSTRUCTIONS

1. To make the tea blend, in a medium bowl, combine the lemon balm, boneset, and marshmallow root. Stir to blend well. Transfer to a clean, airtight container. Dried herbal teas retain potency for up to 1 year if stored correctly.

2. To make a cup of tea, steep 2 teaspoons of the herbal tea blend in the boiling water for 10 to 20 minutes.

Elderflower Lemonade

Makes 2 cups

PREP TIME: *25 to 35 minutes /*
COOK TIME: *10 to 15 minutes*

Creating herbal-infused lemonades in the summer is fun and educational for the whole family. Elderflowers bloom mid- to late June as summer temperatures rise and your desire for thirst-quenching beverages increases. If you're able to harvest fresh elderflowers, they add to the excitement of creating elderflower lemonade—but if not, dried flowers impart just as beautiful of a flavor.

Elderflowers and lemons are a source of bioflavonoids, antioxidants, and vitamin C that work synergistically to ward off seasonal allergies, prevent colds and flus, and act as a diuretic, flushing the kidneys and decreasing water weight.

FOR THE ELDER-FLOWER SIMPLE SYRUP

2 cups water
1 cup dried elderflower, or 2 cups fresh
1 lemon, sliced
2 cups sugar

FOR THE LEMONADE

3 cups cold water
1 cup fresh or bottled lemon juice
½ to 1 cup elderflower simple syrup
Ice, for serving

SUPPLIES

Cutting board and knife
Medium saucepan
Metal sieve
Large pitcher

TO MAKE THE ELDERFLOWER SIMPLE SYRUP

1. In a medium saucepan, combine the water, dried elderflower, and lemon. Bring to a boil over medium-high heat, about 10 to 15 minutes. Remove from the heat. Cover the saucepan, and let infuse for 20 to 30 minutes.

2. Strain the spent flowers from the infusion, and return the infusion to the pan.

3. Add the sugar, and simmer over medium-low heat until reduced by half. Remove from the heat.

TO MAKE THE LEMONADE

4. In a large pitcher, combine the water and lemon juice.

5. Add the simple syrup to taste, and stir well. Refrigerate for 30 minutes to 1 hour, then serve over ice.

Triple Lemon Tea

Makes ¾ cup   **PREP TIME:** *10 minutes*

Lemon verbena is a beautiful and brightly scented plant. It's hard to believe it grows wild in South America. A lemon verbena shrub can grow seven to ten feet tall and has pointed, glossy leaves that are brightly scented of lemons. Lemon verbena tea is supportive for digestive complaints such as indigestion, gas, and constipation and is a source of antioxidants and anti-inflammatory compounds.

The second herb in this triple-herb blend is lemongrass, a source of vitamins A and C. It also comforts the stomach and can be used to treat cold and flu symptoms. This tall aromatic grass is native to Southeast Asia and is used abundantly in Southeast Asian cuisines. Last, lemon balm, native to southern Europe, is a strong antiviral, boosting this blend's effectiveness during illness. Additionally, lemon balm soothes the nerves, which can get aggravated while dealing with illnesses. These three herbs can often be cultivated together in growth zones nine through eleven.

INGREDIENTS

¼ cup dried
  lemon verbena
¼ cup dried lemongrass
¼ cup dried lemon balm
2 tablespoons dried
  ginger (optional)
8 to 12 ounces
  boiling water

SUPPLIES

Medium mixing bowl
Gloves, for blending
  (optional)
Storage container

INSTRUCTIONS

1. To make the tea blend, in a medium bowl, combine the lemon verbena, lemongrass, lemon balm, and ginger (if using). Stir to blend well. Transfer to a clean, airtight container. Dried herbal teas retain potency for up to 1 year if stored correctly.

2. To make a cup of tea, steep 2 tablespoons of the herbal tea blend in the boiling water for 5 to 10 minutes.

Pine Tip Tea

Makes 4 cups   **PREP TIME:** *5 minutes* / **COOK TIME:** *35 minutes*

Although not covered in the herb profiles section, pine bark, tips, and needles were an important medicinal plant to the Native Americans. There are almost fifty different species of pine trees in North America, and you can visit Plants.USDA.gov for the most accurate information for identifying the species in your area.

Most parts of the pine tree can be used medicinally, including the bark, resin, "tops" or "tips," and needles. Poultices were made with pine bark to treat burns, hemorrhoids, ulcers, and wounds. The resin was a livelihood for some eastern Native tribes, because they would travel from North Carolina to Florida collecting it for turpentine that would be sold and used in prescription medicines in the nineteenth and twentieth centuries. The resin was also chewed as a gum, offering comfort to sore throats, and was made into salves to treat sore muscles and joints.

Pine tops or tips are the new growth at the end of a branch and carry much of the sap and vitamin C. These tips can be harvested and dried and used to treat colds and respiratory issues. Often traditional healers would combine them with herbs like mullein, horehound, or goldenrod. Although not as potent as the tops, the needles are also a source of vitamin C.

INGREDIENTS

¼ cup pine tips
4 cups water
Honey or sugar,
  for serving

SUPPLIES

Medium saucepan
Metal sieve

INSTRUCTIONS

1. In a medium saucepan, combine the pine tips and water. Bring to a boil over medium-high heat, about 10 to 15 minutes.

2. Reduce the heat to a simmer. Cook for 20 minutes. Remove from the heat. Strain into a mug.

3. Sweeten with honey to taste.

Spiced Chokecherry Syrup

Makes 2 to 3 cups **PREP TIME:** *5 minutes /* **COOK TIME:** *25 minutes*

Native Americans called these fruit chokecherries because they were so sour they could make you choke. Adding spices and an adequate amount of sugar reduces the sourness, and you end up with a flavorful syrup that can be used as a cold remedy, antidiarrheal, and immune-system booster. High in vitamin C, chokecherry syrup can be used as a preventive against colds and, when taken at the onset of symptoms, to lessen the duration of a cold. Historically, Native Americans used the bark as a heart and blood medicine, so this can also be added to the list of health benefits. The spices not only add a pleasant flavor but also increase the antiviral and antioxidant content of the syrup.

In retail spaces, chokecherries may be labeled as "aronia berries."

INGREDIENTS

1 cup fresh
  chokecherries, or
  ½ cup dried
1 cinnamon stick
5 whole cloves
3 to 5 cardamom pods
2 cups water
½ to 1 cup raw honey

SUPPLIES

Medium saucepan
Metal sieve
Glass jar

INSTRUCTIONS

1. In a medium saucepan, combine the choke-cherries, cinnamon stick, cloves, cardamom, and water. Simmer over medium heat until the liquid has reduced by half. Remove from the heat. Let cool to room temperature.

2. Strain the mixture over a glass jar.

3. Add the honey to taste. Label the jar, and store in the refrigerator for 1 month.

Winterberry Tea

Makes 2 cups   **PREP TIME:** *5 minutes* / **COOK TIME:** *20 minutes*

This tea is a marriage of berries that are foraged early to late fall and offer a punch of immune-boosting properties and so much more! Elderberries gain their rich purple color from the antioxidant anthocyanin. Anthocyanins are a class of flavonoids that have antioxidant effects, meaning they fight free radicals that accumulate in the body and cause aging and oxidative stress. This type of stress increases inflammation, degrades cellular health, and opens the door to illness. Rose hips support the cellular structure of the skin due to their high content of collagen-boosting vitamin C. This false fruit of rose bushes go beyond that, though, also relieving pain, reducing cholesterol, and aiding in digestion. In addition to being an antioxidant source, juniper berries add antibacterial support to this supercharged winter tea. Honeybush adds body to this tea blend and contributes antioxidants and the minerals calcium, iron, copper, and zinc.

INGREDIENTS

½ **cup elderberries**
½ **cup rose hips**
½ **cup honeybush tea**
¼ **cup juniper berries**
¼ **cup rose petals**
A variety of aromatic herbs: star anise, fennel, cinnamon, and ginger
10 ounces water

SUPPLIES

Medium mixing bowl
Gloves, for blending (optional)
Storage container
Small saucepan

INSTRUCTIONS

1. To make the tea blend, in a medium mixing bowl, combine the elderberries, rose hips, honeybush, juniper berries, and rose petals. Stir to blend well. Transfer to a clean, airtight container. Dried herbal teas retain potency for up to 1 year if stored correctly.

2. To make a cup of tea, in a small saucepan, combine 2 tablespoons of the tea blend with the water.

3. Add aromatics if you choose. Cover the pan, and simmer for at least 20 minutes. Remove from the heat. Strain and enjoy!

Wild Violet Sugar

Makes 2 cups

PREP TIME: *20 minutes, plus overnight to dry the flowers*

In the book *Plants Have So Much to Give Us, All We Have to Do Is Ask*, the author, Mary Siisip Geniusz, says, "Violet flowers of spring are just for show. Or perhaps they are just the violets' way of showing their virtues with the rest of creation, as their ancestors were told to do in the beginning time by Creator." She is referring to the fact that violet flowers make their way to the surface even before bee season and aren't necessary for reproduction but do offer us pleasure. The flowers and leaves are a source of nutrition and can be eaten raw or cooked, together or on their own. They make for a beautiful addition to confections, omelets, salads, and even butters. Violet flowers and leaves are a rich source of vitamins A and C, and this plant can be used medicinally for its decongestant and gentle laxative benefits. The best way to consume wild violets as medicine is by making a syrup and taking a teaspoon at a time as needed. This recipe will allow you to preserve and store your violet flowers and easily create a syrup when needed. You can also use this violet-infused syrup in your baking or as a sweet topping.

INGREDIENTS

**1 cup fresh
violet flowers**

**2 cups organic
white sugar**

**2 teaspoons grated
lemon zest**

SUPPLIES

**Food processor
or blender**

Storage container

INSTRUCTIONS

1. Let the flowers dry overnight.

2. Put the flowers, sugar, and lemon zest in a food processor or blender. Pulse until well incorporated. Transfer to a clean, airtight container. Label with the date of preparation, and use within 3 months.

3. To make a violet syrup, in a saucepan, combine sugar and water in a ratio of 2-to-1. Simmer until reduced by half. Remove from the heat.

Constipation-Relief Pastilles

Makes 6 pastilles   **PREP TIME:** *10 minutes*

Herbal pastilles are a blend of finely powdered herbs mixed with honey to create a thick paste that can be rolled into balls. This method of consuming medicinal herbs is best used to cover the taste of bitter herbs and is especially helpful for highly mucilaginous herbs that may goop up in the presence of water, such as slippery elm.

Slippery elm is one of the plants used by Native Americans for its soothing, laxative properties in addition to cascara sagrada. It was used by the Yurok Tribe of California, Swinomish Tribe of Washington, and Flathead Tribe of Montana for its ability to gently move the bowels. Harvesting was done carefully by removing bark from its main trunk or removing a small single limb. Today, according to United Plant Savers, cascara sagrada growth is in decline due to overharvesting and the alteration of its natural habitat due to fire suppression.

INGREDIENTS

2 tablespoons powdered slippery elm

1 tablespoon powdered cascara sagrada

½ tablespoon ginger powder

3 tablespoons ground cinnamon, plus more for rolling

1½ tablespoons honey

SUPPLIES

Small mixing bowl
Microwave-safe bowl
Spatula
Storage container

INSTRUCTIONS

1. In a small mixing bowl, combine the slippery elm, cascara sagrada, ginger, and cinnamon. Stir until blended well.

2. Put the honey in a microwave-safe bowl, and microwave on high for 10 seconds, or until runny.

3. Slowly add the warm honey to the powdered herbs, then blend well. You're aiming for a paste consistency that can be rolled into small balls.

4. Roll the pastilles in cinnamon to dry the outside. Store in an airtight container in the refrigerator for up to 6 months.

Ground Ivy Respiratory Syrup

Makes 4 cups

PREP TIME: *5 minutes, plus 1 hour to steep /*
COOK TIME: *40 minutes*

Ground ivy is an invasive perennial that was brought to North America from Europe and found a home in the Native American apothecary. This combination of medicinal plants works together to decrease inflammation and infection of the ears, nose, and throat.

INGREDIENTS

5 cups water
1 to 2 cups honey
  or sugar
1 cup ground ivy
A few thyme sprigs
¼ cup marshmallow
  root or licorice root
1 large slice dried
  reishi (optional)

SUPPLIES

Medium saucepan
Metal sieve or funnel
Sanitized
  storage container
Cheesecloth

INSTRUCTIONS

1. In a medium saucepan, combine the water, honey, ground ivy, thyme, marshmallow root, and mushroom (if using). Bring to a boil over medium-high heat, about 10 to 15 minutes.

2. Reduce the heat to a simmer. Let the mixture reduce by half. Remove from the heat. Let continue steeping for up to 1 hour.

3. Place a sieve or funnel over a sanitized container, cover with two layers of cheesecloth, and strain. Pick up the cloth in a bundle, and carefully squeeze.

4. For every 1 cup of decocted liquid, add ½ cup of honey or sugar. If using honey, pour honey into the warm decoction, and stir until completely dissolved. If using sugar, return the decocted liquid to the pan, add sugar, and simmer gently until completely dissolved. Remove from the heat. Let cool before storing.

5. Using a funnel, pour the syrup into the sanitized container. Seal well, label, and store in the refrigerator for up to 3 weeks.

Honeysuckle Cough Syrup

Makes 2 cups   **PREP TIME:** *25 minutes* / **COOK TIME:** *15 minutes*

Honeysuckle is a slow-growing vine usually found in open woodlands and borders. The flower is now the most common part of the plant used for medicinal purposes, but the Native Americans also used the leaves as a purgative before ceremonies and the bark for homesickness. Today, the honeysuckle flower is used as a respiratory aid because of its ability to thin fluids like mucus so it can be coughed up with ease. It is also used as a kidney aid, increasing urine production. Honeysuckle also tones the tissues, preventing water loss, and is an antispasmodic, supportive for those with asthma. Mullein is a demulcent herb and balances the dryness of honeysuckle, lending a soothing effect to the respiratory tissues but also working as an expectorant, moving excess fluid out of the lungs and chest. Ginger works as a natural decongestant and antihistamine. It is also a powerful antiviral and antibacterial herb that strengthens the immune system.

INGREDIENTS

1 cup fresh
  honeysuckle flowers
1 or 2 fresh
  mullein leaves
1 (1-inch) piece ginger,
  roughly chopped
2 cups water
1 cup honey
Juice of 1 lemon

SUPPLIES

Cutting board and knife
Medium saucepan
Metal sieve
  and cheesecloth
Sanitized storage jar

INSTRUCTIONS

1. In a medium saucepan, combine the honeysuckle, mullein, ginger, and water. Simmer over medium heat until reduced by half. Remove from the heat. Let cool for at least 20 minutes.

2. Strain the mixture over a sanitized container.

3. Stir in the honey and lemon juice until fully incorporated. Label the container, and store in the refrigerator for up to 4 weeks.

Wild Ramp Cough Syrup

Makes 2 cups   **PREP TIME:** *5 minutes* / **COOK TIME:** *30 minutes*

Wild ramps are in the allium or onion family and grow in the understory of forests from the Dakotas throughout the eastern states to North Carolina. Ramps are an especially popular spring food in the Appalachian states, the original home of the Cherokee peoples. Southeastern woodland tribes like the Cherokee consumed ramps to treat coughs and colds, made ramp poultices to heal insect stings, and used the juice of these wild leeks to treat earaches.

Ramps are a slow-growing cultivar of the onion family that is at risk of being overharvested. For this reason, store-bought onions may be the best option for this recipe. The sulfur-containing amino acid allicin is antibacterial, giving the onion the nickname "nature's antibiotic." Onions also contain essential oils, flavonoids, and nutrients that are anti-inflammatory. They thin mucus while activating the chest and stimulating a cough that is productive, helping the body expel congestion. In addition to being soothing to throat tissues, honey adds even more antibacterial power to this immune-boosting cough syrup.

INGREDIENTS

1 cup sliced onions
2 garlic cloves
**2 tablespoons freshly
  squeezed lemon juice**
2 cups honey

SUPPLIES

Cutting board and knife
Medium saucepan
**Widemouthed glass
  jar, sanitized**

INSTRUCTIONS

1. In a medium saucepan, combine the onions, garlic, lemon juice, and honey. Warm over low heat for at least 30 minutes. Remove from the heat. Pour into a sanitized glass jar. Store in the refrigerator for up to 3 months.

2. To use the syrup, take 1 to 2 teaspoons as needed.

Potent Detox Tea with Chaparral

Makes 1¼ cups   **PREP TIME:** *10 minutes*

This tea blend is a strong mix of detoxifying herbs, most of which you have read about or will read about throughout this book, apart from chaparral. Also known as creosote bush, chaparral is native to the lower western states. Tribes that historically used this medicinal plant include the Cahuilla, Isleta, Paiute, and Shoshone. Documented uses by the Native Americans include cancer treatment, cold remedy, and respiratory aid. It is also used to help with wound healing, stomach discomfort, menstrual cramps, and swollen joints. Chaparral is a bitter-tasting herb that is tempered by the other herbs in the recipe. Burdock, dandelion, ginger, and red clover also support the organs that assimilate nutrients and remove waste, such as the liver, kidneys, and lymph nodes. The ginger is a nice accompaniment to enhance flavor and is known to calm inflammation that may get exacerbated from the amount of detoxification at work. This is a tea you may consume for short periods of time to enhance a cleansing diet.

INGREDIENTS

¼ **cup dried
  burdock root**
¼ **cup dried
  dandelion root**
¼ **cup dried
  chaparral leaves**
¼ **cup red clover**
¼ **cup dried ginger**
**8 to 12 ounces
  boiling water**

SUPPLIES

Medium mixing bowl
**Gloves, for blending
  (optional)**
Storage container

INSTRUCTIONS

1. To make the tea blend, in a medium bowl, combine the burdock, dandelion, chaparral, clover, and ginger. Stir to blend well. Transfer to a clean, airtight container. Dried herbal teas retain potency for up to 1 year if stored correctly.

2. To make a cup of tea, steep 2 teaspoons of the herbal tea blend in the boiling water for 5 minutes.

Dandelion Bitters Tincture

Makes 2 cups   **PREP TIME:** *20 minutes, plus at least 4 weeks to infuse*

Many of the Indigenous herbs listed are categorized as "blood medicine." It is believed that these herbs increase the quality of the blood by supporting the liver in detoxification while supplying the blood with a concentrated nutrition in the form of vitamins, minerals, and trace elements. In modern herbalism, these herbs are called "alteratives," or blood purifiers. These bitter herbs tone systems, neutralize acids, dry excess moisture, and stimulate secretion of gastric juices that aid the gallbladder and liver in digesting and assimilating fats.

Dandelion leaves and the root are by far one of the most popular bitter herbs that can be easily foraged. The Algonquin, Cherokee, and Haudenosaunee are among the several peoples that consumed dandelion in some form to restore the blood, recognizing its usage for anemia, skin sores, liver spots, and puffiness.

INGREDIENTS

½ cup dandelion root

½ cup dandelion leaves

2 tablespoons fennel seeds

2 tablespoons orange peel (with rind)

2 cups 80-proof alcohol

SUPPLIES

Clean glass jar with lid

Metal sieve

Storage container

Funnel

Dropper bottles

INSTRUCTIONS

1. In a glass jar, combine the dandelion root, dandelion leaves, fennel seeds, and orange peel.

2. Add enough alcohol to cover by 1 inch. Seal the jar tightly, and label. Place in a cool, shady spot, and gently shake every few days for 4 to 6 weeks.

3. To strain, place a sieve over an open container, and pour in the tincture extract. Gently press the plant material to release all fluid.

4. Using a funnel, pour the fluid into dropper bottles. Alcohol is one of the most effective preservatives, meaning tinctures produced in this manner generally have a shelf life of at least 1 year, and sometimes up to 3 years.

Fireweed Simple Syrup

Makes 2 cups   **PREP TIME:** *5 minutes* / **COOK TIME:** *40 minutes*

Simple syrups are easy to make and fun to add to teas, lattes, and spritzers. Infusing them with flowers like fireweed, violets, and rose petals adds beauty as well as nutritional and medicinal benefits. Fireweed is packed with antioxidants and can lessen the burden of inflammation on the body. Nutritionally, it is a source of vitamins A and C. Fireweed-leaf tea has an affinity for the digestive system, offering toning benefits and increasing good gut flora. This syrup can be used to sweeten the slight bitterness of infused leaves for a complete healing experience.

Tips for creating beautiful simple syrups:

- Infuse flowers in water until their color has faded, and remove them before adding sugar.

- Use white sugar if you want to maintain the pure color of the flowers.

- Reduce the water-sugar mixture enough to create a thickened syrup.

- A 1-to-1 water-sugar ratio is ideal for longer preservation.

INGREDIENTS

2 cups water
1 cup fresh fireweed
  flowers, or
  ½ cup dried
2 cups white sugar

INSTRUCTIONS

1. In a medium saucepan, bring the water to a boil over medium-high heat.

2. Reduce the heat to low. Add the flowers, cover the pan, and simmer for 5 minutes. Remove from the heat. Let sit for 20 minutes.

3. Strain the flowers, and return the infused water to the pan.

SUPPLIES

Medium saucepan
Metal sieve
**Sanitized glass
  storage container**

4. Add the sugar, and bring to a boil over medium heat. Let the mixture reduce by half. Remove from the heat. Let cool, then transfer the syrup to a sanitized glass container. Label, then store in the refrigerator for up to 4 weeks.

Quick Pickled Cattails

Makes 8 cups

PREP TIME: *15 minutes, plus at least 1 week to pickle /*
COOK TIME: *15 minutes*

Pickling cattails is not much different from pickling any other type of vegetable. In this recipe, you can mix and match vegetables or use only cattails. Cattails are a source of vitamins and minerals as well as soluble and insoluble fiber. Consuming them regularly can improve digestion, blood sugar, and skin health.

INGREDIENTS

**1 pound cattails, or a
  mixture of cattails and
  other vegetables**
**3 cups distilled white or
  apple cider vinegar**
3 cups water
**5 tablespoons
  pickling salt**
**1 tablespoon
  sugar (optional)**
1 bay leaf
**2 sprigs any herbs
  (optional)**

SUPPLIES

Cutting board and knife
**2 (1-pint) widemouthed
  jars with lids,
  sanitized**
Large saucepan

INSTRUCTIONS

1. Clean the cattails, and cut away at the tough ends and exterior until you reach the soft heart or middle.

2. Place the cattails standing up in two sanitized jars.

3. In a large saucepan, combine the vinegar, water, salt, and sugar (if using). Bring to a boil over medium-high heat. Cook until the salt and sugar have dissolved. Remove from the heat. Pour over the cattails, leaving a ½-inch headspace.

4. Tuck in the bay leaf and any other fresh or dried herbs. Seal the jar, and shake well to incorporate. Refrigerate for 1 week before enjoying.

Roasted Burdock Root and Beets

Makes 3 cups

PREP TIME: *20 minutes /*
COOK TIME: *55 minutes to 1 hour 20 minutes*

Burdock root is a source of antioxidants (quercetin), minerals (potassium, magnesium, and selenium), and vitamins B, C, E, and K. This taproot also contains 45 percent inulin fiber, feeding gut flora, strengthening the microbiome, and allowing for better digestion.

Native Americans believed burdock purified the blood, and through its ability to support the liver and kidneys, this root offers a cleansing effect by moving toxins out of the body and supporting clearer skin and hormone balance. Beets also have a liver-supporting nutritional profile of iron, B vitamins, and a compound called betaine that is especially helpful in the elimination of toxins. This nutritionally dense combination of beets and burdock increases the health of the liver, gallbladder, and heart.

INGREDIENTS

1 cup diced
   burdock root
2 cups diced beets
2 garlic cloves, chopped
2 tablespoons olive oil
Salt
Freshly ground
   black pepper
2 tablespoons coconut
   aminos (optional)

SUPPLIES

Knife and cutting board
Strainer
Small saucepan
Large mixing bowl
Baking sheet

INSTRUCTIONS

1. Soak the burdock root in cold water for 10 minutes. Drain, rinse, and transfer to a small saucepan.

2. Fill the saucepan with water, and bring to a boil over medium-high heat. Boil for 20 to 30 minutes, or until the burdock root has partially cooked. Remove from the heat.

3. Meanwhile, preheat the oven to 425°F.

4. In a large mixing bowl, combine the boiled burdock root, beets, garlic, and olive oil. Season with salt and pepper. Toss well.

5. Evenly distribute the vegetables over a sheet pan.

6. Transfer the sheet pan to the oven, and roast for 30 to 45 minutes, or until tender. Remove from the oven.

7. Add the coconut aminos (if using).

Mullein Flower Ear Oil

Makes 2 ounces

PREP TIME: *5 minutes, plus at least 10 hours to infuse /*
COOK TIME: *40 minutes*

Mullein is an aggressive-growing biennial, meaning it goes to seed only every other year and produces seeds that have a high rate of germination, which reproduce several plants that year. Mullein grows in abandoned lots, along the roadways, on the sides of mountains, and in rocky soils. The leaves are stemless, growing directly from the ground, and can get as large as twenty inches long and five inches wide. On its year of reproduction, a large erect stem will grow from the center of the plant, getting very tall and producing small yellow flowers about three-quarters of an inch in size with five delicate petals. The leaves are known for their respiratory benefits and the flowers for their anti-inflammatory effect in cases of infection. The garlic in this formula offers antiseptic properties in the form of organic sulfur. Wild garlic was also used as ear medicine by the Cherokee, as well as a remedy against edema and high blood pressure.

INGREDIENTS

2 ounces olive oil
1 garlic clove,
   thinly sliced
2 tablespoons
   mullein flowers

SUPPLIES

Cutting board and knife
Small saucepan
Metal sieve
Storage container
Small funnel
Dropper bottles

INSTRUCTIONS

1. In a small saucepan, combine the oil, garlic, and mullein. Warm over low heat for at least 40 minutes. Remove from the heat. Cover the pan, and let infuse for 10 to 12 hours.

2. Using a metal sieve, strain the herbs from the oil over a container.

3. Funnel the oil into dropper bottles. Store in a dark cabinet for up to 1 month. Warm the oil before dropping 2 to 4 drops in the affected ear.

Healthy Energy Herbal Balls

Makes 12 balls   **PREP TIME:** *30 minutes*

These nut-butter balls include beneficial nutritive and herb powders that support energy production, cellular health, and even reduced levels of cholesterol. Guarana, a plant native to South America, has seeds that are ground and brewed like coffee beans and contain a trace number of vitamins, minerals, and antioxidants that help support the heart. The Sateré-Mawé Tribe created smoking "sticks" with guarana seeds by grinding the seeds up in a mortar and pestle, blending this powder with water, and rolling the mixture into sticks to dry in the sun. Spirulina has been shown to lower "bad" cholesterol, and studies show cacao can increase "good" cholesterol.

INGREDIENTS

1 cup tahini
½ cup almond butter
½ cup honey
3 tablespoons raw cacao powder, plus more for rolling
2 tablespoons guarana powder
2 tablespoons spirulina powder
2 teaspoons ground cinnamon, plus more for rolling
¼ cup crushed raw cacao nibs

SUPPLIES

Large mixing bowl
Small mixing bowl
Strong mixing spatula
Storage container

INSTRUCTIONS

1. In a large bowl, mix together the tahini, almond butter, and honey.

2. In a small bowl, combine the cacao powder, guarana powder, spirulina powder, and cinnamon. Mix to blend well.

3. Slowly add the powder blend to the wet ingredients, blending until the consistency becomes thick.

4. Blend in the crushed cacao nibs for texture. Roll the mixture into balls 1 inch in diameter.

5. If desired, you can roll the balls in cinnamon or cacao powder to dry the outside.

6. Refrigerate the balls in a clean, airtight container for up to 6 weeks.

Strengthening Iron Tonic

Makes 1 quart   **PREP TIME:** *5 minutes* / **COOK TIME:** *2 to 3 hours*

This recipe can be used as a plant-based replacement for iron supplements, as well as a source of other minerals such as calcium, magnesium, silica, and potassium. Molasses and apricots are amazing sources of iron and add a nice sweetness to this tonic, and the orange peel and rose hips supply vitamin C, increasing the bioavailability of iron. Taking an ounce of this formula daily can increase energy and vitality.

INGREDIENTS

12 cups water
**⅓ cup dried
 eleuthero root**
⅓ cup dried rose hips
⅓ cup dried apricots
**1 (1-inch) slice organic
 orange peel**
**½ cup dried
 nettle leaves**
½ cup dried oat straw
**1 cup blackstrap
 molasses**

SUPPLIES

Large pot
Large spoon or spatula
Metal sieve
Large mixing bowl
Cheesecloth
Glass jar or bottle

INSTRUCTIONS

1. In a large pot, combine the water, eleuthero, rose hips, and apricots.

2. Add the orange peel, and partially cover the pot. Bring the mixture to a simmer over medium heat. Cook for 2 to 3 hours, or until reduced by half. Remove from the heat.

3. Stir in the nettles, oat straw, and molasses. Cover the pot, and let sit overnight.

4. Place a metal sieve over a large bowl, cover with two or three layers of cheesecloth, and pour the herb mixture over the top. Pull up the corners of the cheesecloth to squeeze out excess liquid.

5. Pour the herbal tonic into a glass jar or bottle, and store in the refrigerator for up to 1 month.

Yaupon Tea or "Black Drink"

Makes 2 cups   **PREP TIME:** *30 minutes*

Yaupon tea, also called "cassina" by the Timucua people and "black drink" by the Spanish explorers, has been sipped for centuries among the Indigenous in purifying ceremonies and for its uplifting, energetic qualities. A cup of yaupon tea contains an average of 25 milligrams of caffeine, which is less than a cup of coffee. It also contains the positive compounds theobromine and theacrine, which offer a mental and emotional boost. Like green tea, but without the risk of overbrewing causing a bitter flavor, yaupon tea contains an ample number of antioxidants that slow the rate of aging and promote cellular health.

Yaupon tea was a popular beverage in the fifteenth and sixteenth centuries, but grew out of favor by the 1800s, except among the Cherokee people, who still consumed it for ceremonial purposes. By the 1900s, yaupon faded into obscurity. In recent years, yaupon's popularity has returned with a surge of brands and even tea shops highlighting this beautiful southeastern shrub. Yaupon leaves have a grassy, earthy, orange-tinged flavor and are best roasted for optimum enjoyment.

INGREDIENTS

**1 cup yaupon
  holly leaves**
**8 to 10 ounces
  boiling water**

SUPPLIES

Baking sheet
Cutting board and knife
Storage container
**Infuser, fillable tea
  bags, or metal sieve**

INSTRUCTIONS

1. Preheat the oven to 350°F.

2. Put the yaupon leaves on a baking sheet.

3. Transfer the baking sheet to the oven, and roast the leaves until they turn your desired shade of brown. The darker the leaves, the richer your brew will be. Remove from the oven. Let cool.

4. Once cool, chop the leaves into smaller pieces. Store in a clean, airtight container for up to 2 years.

5. To make a cup of tea, infuse 2 teaspoons of yaupon leaves in the boiling water for 5 minutes before serving.

Milkweed Seed Bombs

**Makes 15 to
20 seed bombs**

PREP TIME: *30 minutes, plus at least 24 hours
to air-dry*

According to Daniel Moerman, the author of *Native American Medicinal Plants*, there were at least twenty-four different milkweed species that were used by tribes throughout North America. The milkweed plant is the only plant monarch butterflies lay their eggs on, making them critical for the survival of the species, and the leaves are also their primary food source. Unfortunately, the monarch population has experienced a decline due to air pollution, climate change, pesticides, and loss of habitat. Several species of milkweed exist, but only about 25 percent of them are known to be hosts for monarch species, so before picking your seeds, visit Plants.USDA.gov to learn which species thrive in your area.

INGREDIENTS

1 cup all-natural clay
1 cup seed-starting
 soil mix
½ cup water, plus more
 as needed
1 teaspoon
 milkweed seeds

SUPPLIES

Large mixing bowl
Toothpick
Baking sheet
Parchment paper

INSTRUCTIONS

1. In a large bowl, combine the clay, soil, and water. Mix until a cookie-dough consistency is achieved and the mixture is sticky enough that the clay and soil adhere. Add more water as needed.

2. Roll the mixture into 1-inch balls.

3. Using a toothpick, poke 15 to 20 holes into each ball, and place seeds into each hole. Roll each ball again until smooth.

4. Put prepared balls on a baking sheet, and let them air-dry for 24 to 48 hours.

5. Prior to forecasted rain, throw the balls into open fields and lots to give them an opportunity to grow.

Catnip Glycerite

Makes 1 cup

PREP TIME: *15 minutes, plus at least 4 weeks to macerate*

A glycerite is a tincture made with glycerin as the solvent rather than alcohol to extract or preserve the medicinal properties of an herb. Although not as potent as alcohol tinctures, glycerites are especially good for fussy children and people intolerant of alcohol due to allergies or addiction. The dosage for adults is usually thirty to sixty drops taken three times a day with water. Children ages nine to twelve years old can usually tolerate thirty drops, but for younger children, decrease the number of drops by six to ten depending on the size of the child. Catnip is calming to the nervous system, and it can also ease digestion by supporting the release of uncomfortable gas such as colic in infants.

INGREDIENTS

¼ cup distilled water

¾ cup glycerin

1 tablespoon dried catnip, or ¼ cup fresh, finely chopped

SUPPLIES

Measuring cup

8-ounce jar, with tight-fitting lid

Dull knife or chopstick

Metal sieve

Storage container

Cheesecloth

Funnel

Dropper bottles or jar

INSTRUCTIONS

1. In a measuring cup, combine the water and glycerin. Stir until well blended.

2. Put the catnip in the jar. Using a dull knife or chopstick, press down on the plant material as you pour the water-glycerin mixture over it, releasing air bubbles, until full. Seal the jar, label, and set in a cool, dark spot to macerate for 4 to 6 weeks.

3. To decant: Place a sieve over a container, and cover with two or three layers of cheesecloth. Pour the jar contents into the sieve. Once done, lift the corners of the cheesecloth to create a bundle, and squeeze gently to release the remainder of the glycerite.

4. Using a funnel, pour the contents into dropper bottles, a jar, or other long-term storage containers. Label and date accordingly. Glycerin tinctures typically expire after 1 year.

Goldenrod Salve

Makes 1 cup

PREP TIME: *5 minutes /*
COOK TIME: *1 hour 55 minutes*

Salves combine a plant-infused oil, solid oil, and beeswax to create a solid formula that travels easier than an infused oil in liquid form. Once you learn the basic measurements for making salves, they become easy to create with different plants healing various ailments. Goldenrod is used in this recipe for its anti-inflammatory properties and can be used on sore muscles, arthritis, burns, scrapes, and other minor skin irritations. If using freshly harvested goldenrod tops, make sure to allow them to dry a few days before infusing into oil.

INGREDIENTS

1 cup coconut oil or
   olive oil
½ cup dried goldenrod
1 ounce
   beeswax pellets

SUPPLIES

Double boiler
Metal sieve
Cheesecloth
Storage containers

INSTRUCTIONS

1. Place the oil and goldenrod in the top of a double boiler.

2. Bring water to a simmer in the lower part of the double boiler over medium heat. Let the herbs and oil infuse for 30 minutes to 1 hour. Remove from the heat.

3. Using a sieve and cheesecloth, strain the goldenrod over a container. Make sure to squeeze the excess oil from your spent herbs and compost them.

4. Return the oil to the double boiler, and add the beeswax. Warm over low heat until the oil and beeswax have fully combined. Remove from the heat. You can check your mixture for solidity by putting a spoonful on a plate and putting it in the freezer for 5 to 10 minutes. If the mixture is too soft for your liking, add more beeswax 1 teaspoon at a time.

5. Pour the mixture into containers while hot, and let solidify before sealing to avoid condensation. Salve expiration times vary from 3 months to 1 year, depending on the volatility of the oils and the amount of beeswax. Look for signs of aging such as separation, mold, or an off-putting smell.

Gas-Relief Tea

Makes 1 cup   **PREP TIME:** *5 minutes*

The fermentation of foods within the digestive system is the main culprit of gas. Preventive measures can be taken, and herbs are highly effective at calming the symptoms. To prevent gas, practice healthy habits like slowing down before and during your meals, chewing sufficiently, watching how much you consume, and choosing whole foods as much as possible. However, when gas happens anyway, aromatic, carminative (flatulence-reducing) herbs are your go-to to calm the belly rumbles. Peppermint and lemon balm both have a cooling effect on the digestive system and effectively quell stomach spasms. Chamomile is especially welcome when stomach distress is due to stress or anxiety. When brewed for an extended amount of time, chamomile will be slightly bitter, stimulating digestive enzymes within the digestive system. Fennel seed is well-known as a warming carminative herb, and it is also antimicrobial, antifungal, and anti-inflammatory.

INGREDIENTS

¼ cup dried
  peppermint leaves
¼ cup dried lemon
  balm leaves
¼ cup chamomile
  flowers
¼ cup fennel seeds
8 to 12 ounces
  boiling water

SUPPLIES

Medium mixing bowl
Gloves, for blending
  (optional)
Storage container

INSTRUCTIONS

1. To make the tea blend, in a medium bowl, combine the peppermint, lemon balm, chamomile, and fennel. Stir until well blended. Transfer to a clean, airtight container. Dried herbal teas retain potency for up to 1 year if stored correctly.

2. To make a cup of tea, steep 2 teaspoons of the herbal tea blend in the boiling water for 10 to 20 minutes.

Stress-Induced Headache Tincture

Makes 1 cup   **PREP TIME:** *20 minutes, plus at least 4 weeks to infuse*

When choosing herbs to heal a headache, it is important to know what's causing the pain in the first place. Some reasons for headaches include food intolerances, hormonal imbalances, migraines, stress, and tension. This formula concentrates on headaches that are brought on by stress and tension in the neck and shoulders. Feverfew is the herbalist's go-to as a preventive for those who experience head pain regularly from stress or migraines. Chamomile calms the spirit and acts as an anti-inflammatory working throughout the body. Lemon balm, especially fresh, has deeply permeating essential oils. This formula can offer an uplifting effect when you are anxious from pain. Blue vervain quickly releases tension, especially in the neck and shoulders, improving the mood and stimulating the release of dopamine and serotonin, which are "feel-good" hormones. This tincture is best used as a preventive during especially stressful times and upon the first onset of pain.

INGREDIENTS

¼ cup dried feverfew
¼ cup dried chamomile
¼ cup dried lemon balm
2 tablespoons
  blue vervain
1½ cups
  80-proof alcohol

SUPPLIES

4-cup glass jar
Metal sieve
Storage container
Funnel
Dropper bottles

INSTRUCTIONS

1. Put the feverfew, chamomile, lemon balm, and blue vervain in a 4-cup glass jar.

2. Add enough alcohol to cover by 1 inch. Seal the jar tightly, label, and put in a cool, shady spot. Gently shake every few days for 4 to 6 weeks.

3. To strain, place a sieve over an open container, and pour in the tincture extract. Gently press the plant material to release all fluid.

4. Using a funnel, pour the fluid into dropper bottles. Store away from light for up to 3 years.

Angelica Elixir

Makes 2½ cups   **PREP TIME:** *25 minutes, plus at least 3 weeks to infuse*

Native Americans used angelica root as a cold and cough remedy, for intestinal block-ages, and for bronchitis. The bitterness of angelica root increases the production of stomach acids and is especially helpful for sluggish digestion, stimulating appetite and moving intestinal gas out of the system by way of a bactericidal effect on the GI tract.

   Like angelica root, the seeds in this elixir are carminatives that also ease digestive discomfort. It is worth pointing out that this formulation can be incredibly support-ive if the digestive issues are associated with premenstrual symptoms, because anise seeds and coriander seeds are sources of calcium and magnesium, which aid in the relaxation of smooth muscles, including the uterus and intestines. Cinnamon adds warmth to this formula and has anti-inflammatory properties.

INGREDIENTS

2 tablespoons
   anise seeds
2 tablespoons
   coriander seeds
1 teaspoon
   fennel seeds
1 cinnamon stick
2 ounces dried
   angelica root
Peel and juice of
   ½ orange
2 cups brandy
¼ to ½ cup honey

INSTRUCTIONS

1. Using a mortar and pestle, crush the anise, cori-ander, fennel, and cinnamon. Transfer to a 4-cup widemouthed jar.

2. Add the angelica root, orange peel, and orange juice.

3. Pour the brandy over to cover completely. Seal the jar, label, and set in a cool, dark spot. Gently shake every few days for 3 to 4 weeks.

SUPPLIES

Mortar and pestle

**4-cup widemouthed jar
with lid, sanitized**

**Metal sieve
or cheesecloth**

Storage container

4. Strain the mixture through a sieve over a container.

5. Add the honey to taste. Tightly seal the container, and store in a cabinet for up to 1 year.

Saw Palmetto Tincture

Makes 2 cups · **PREP TIME:** *15 minutes, plus at least 4 weeks to infuse*

Saw palmetto berries are used in herbal formulas that support men's reproductive health. This herb may be recommended by an herbalist to help treat prostate enlargement, dull pain in the prostate area, and weakened sexual desire. Saw palmetto can also be an herbal aid for women dealing with hair loss due to excess testosterone, because it may inhibit the excess production of this hormone in women. Corn silk refers to the soft silky strands found inside the corn husk and outside the cob. These strands have been used by Indigenous tribes for centuries to support urinary and kidney health; in this formula, the strands are used because of their ability to promote adequate urine flow, also aiding the health of the prostate gland.

INGREDIENTS

1 cup dried saw
  palmetto berries
½ cup dried corn silk
2 cups 80-proof alcohol

SUPPLIES

4-cup glass jar
Metal sieve
Storage container
Funnel
Dropper bottles

INSTRUCTIONS

1. Put the saw palmetto berries and corn silk in a 4-cup glass jar.

2. Add enough alcohol to cover by 1 inch. Seal the jar tightly, and label. Put in a cool, shady spot, and gently shake every few days for 4 to 6 weeks.

3. To strain, place a sieve over an open container, and pour in the tincture extract. Gently press the plant material to release all fluid.

4. Using a funnel, pour the fluid into dropper bottles. Label, and store in a cool, shady spot for up to 3 years.

Chaga-Infused Instant Latte

Serves 1   **PREP TIME:** *10 minutes*

Chaga mushroom has a similar flavor to coffee and can be used in lieu of or in addition to coffee to increase the nutritional content. An antioxidant powerhouse, chaga can fight the free radicals that speed up the rate of aging. Chaga also stimulates white blood cells, helping ward off viral and bacterial infections. Chaga is referred to as an immune modulator because it adapts to the needs of the immune system; sometimes this means stimulating the system, whereas other times it means calming the system. Chaga also has anti-inflammatory properties, supports heart health, supports healthy blood sugar, and improves stress response.

Chaga is a slow-growing mushroom that is found on the bark of birch trees growing in Alaska, Canada, and other northern regions. Because of the limitations of its growth, it is in danger of being overharvested. This means it is best to look for a product that has been propagated for the purpose of consumption rather than being wild-harvested.

INGREDIENTS

1 teaspoon
  chaga powder

1 teaspoon instant
  coffee (optional)

½ teaspoon
  vanilla extract

1 cup hot water

¼ cup milk, or
  2 tablespoons
  whipping cream

Sprinkle of ground
  cinnamon or
  nutmeg (optional)

SUPPLIES

Blender
Mug

INSTRUCTIONS

1. Put the chaga powder, instant coffee (if using), vanilla, water, and milk in a blender. Blend well for 2 minutes. Pour into a mug.

2. Sprinkle with cinnamon (if using). Sip and cozy up!

Elderberry Syrup

Makes 4 cups

PREP TIME: *10 minutes* / **COOK TIME:** *1 hour 50 minutes*

Research supports Indigenous peoples' belief that elderberries are an effective remedy for respiratory ailments. A source of antioxidants and vitamins, elderberry syrup has the ability to lessen the severity of cold symptoms and aid in recovery. Astragalus is a Chinese herb that has been used for centuries to improve immune function.

INGREDIENTS

**1½ cups
  dried elderberries**
5 cups water
**1 tablespoon
  dried ginger, or
  2 tablespoons fresh**
1 cinnamon stick
**2 tablespoons dried
  astragalus (optional)**
**1 to 2 cups honey
  or sugar**

SUPPLIES

Medium saucepan
Metal sieve or funnel
Cheesecloth
**Sanitized storage
  container**

INSTRUCTIONS

1. In a medium saucepan, combine the elderberries, water, ginger, cinnamon, and astragalus (if using). Bring to a boil over medium-high heat, about 10 to 15 minutes.

2. Reduce the heat to a simmer. Let the mixture reduce by half. Remove from the heat. Continue to steep for up to 1 hour.

3. Place a sieve or funnel over a sanitized container, cover with two layers of cheesecloth, and strain the decocted herbs into the cloth. Pick up the cloth in a bundle, and carefully squeeze.

4. Decide the sweetener ratio: For every 1 cup of decocted liquid, add ½ cup of honey or sugar. If using honey, pour the honey into the warm decoction, and stir until completely dissolved. If using sugar, return the liquid to the pan, add the sugar, and simmer gently until completely dissolved. Remove from the heat. Cool before storing; using the funnel, pour the syrup into the sanitized container.

5. Seal the container well, label, and store in the refrigerator for up to 3 weeks.

Huckleberry-Basil Shrub

Makes 4 cups   **PREP TIME:** *20 minutes, plus 1 week to infuse*

A shrub is a mixture of vinegar, seasonal fruits, and herbs combined with sugar to preserve the year's harvest. Vinegar infusion has been a preservation method for thousands of years and was more available and (currently still is) less expensive than alcohol. Shrub-infused beverages have become popular in recent years and can be mixed with sparkling waters with or without alcohol. They are a delicious way to enjoy the medicinal benefits of many plants and allow for so much creativity. Not only are shrubs fun and delicious, but also each ingredient carries a health benefit; primarily the vinegar supports healthy blood-sugar levels, aiding our own bodies in processing sugars. Both basil and huckleberries are antioxidant-rich foods high in vitamin A, supporting the immune system and eye health.

INGREDIENTS

1 cup huckleberries
1½ cups sugar
2 to 4 fresh basil leaves
1½ cups boiling water
1 cup distilled
  white vinegar

SUPPLIES

4-cup glass jar
Muddler or
  similar utensil
Metal sieve and/or
  cheesecloth
Container

INSTRUCTIONS

1. Put the huckleberries, sugar, and basil in the jar, and muddle (smash together).

2. Cover with the water, and let steep for 10 minutes.

3. Add the vinegar. Refrigerate for at least 1 week to infuse.

4. Strain out the solids over an open container, and pour the liquid back into the jar. Seal and store for up to 4 weeks.

5. To use: Shrubs can be used to make mocktails or cocktails; mix with sparkling water.

Lymph-Mover Tea

Makes 2 cups   **PREP TIME:** *10 minutes*

A vital part of the immune system, the lymphatic system's role is to produce white blood cells, releasing them into the bloodstream so they can fight off bacteria, viruses, fungi, and parasites. It also removes waste products and abnormal cells by way of the lymphatic fluid. Lymph fluid is circulated by way of movement such as exercise and rebounding (trampoline); dry-brushing is an alternative method of lymph-fluid circulation. Herbs can also enhance our lymphatic systems, helping white blood cells get to the areas they are most needed.

Echinacea, burdock, and violet leaves are all lymphatic-supporting herbs used by the Native Americans. Calendula is native to Europe and has been incorporated in Indigenous remedies. This combination of herbs can flush out toxins, decrease congestion, and reduce swollen lymph nodes while increasing the immune system's capacity to work efficiently. Echinacea has been researched enough to prove its efficacy when it comes to stimulating the immune system, fighting infections and healing external wounds and skin problems.

INGREDIENTS

1 cup dried violet leaves
½ cup dried burdock
¼ cup dried echinacea root
¼ cup dried calendula blossoms
8 to 12 ounces boiling water

SUPPLIES

Medium mixing bowl
Gloves, for blending (optional)
Storage container

INSTRUCTIONS

1. To make the tea blend, in a medium bowl, combine the violet leaves, burdock, echinacea, and calendula. Stir to blend well. Transfer to a clean, airtight container. Dried herbal teas retain potency for up to 1 year if stored correctly.

2. To make a cup of tea, steep 2 teaspoons of the herbal tea blend in the water for 5 to 10 minutes.

Strawberry and Hibiscus Shrub

Makes 4 cups   **PREP TIME:** *15 minutes*

It may seem like a surprise that strawberries grow wild in North America, but there are a few varied species growing throughout the continent, and they are referred to as "woodland strawberries" or "wild strawberries." Like corn, wild strawberries were part of traditional Native American diets and were often mentioned in stories passed on through generations. Many Indigenous peoples consider strawberries to be a symbol of blessing, and the Cherokee associate them with love, luck, and happiness. The leaves and roots also played a medicinal role among tribes for stomach disorders and scurvy prevention. They were also used topically on sores as a disinfectant.

This beautiful and tangy mixture of hibiscus and strawberries is abundant in vitamin C and immune-boosting antioxidants. It can be used in a variety of ways and created with your preference of vinegar.

INGREDIENTS

3 cups strawberries
½ cup dried hibiscus
1 cup honey
½ cup balsamic vinegar

SUPPLIES

4-cup widemouthed
  jar, sanitized
Muddler
Blender
Metal sieve and/or
  cheesecloth

INSTRUCTIONS

1. Put the strawberries, hibiscus, and honey in a 4-cup widemouthed jar. Muddle until fully broken down and blended. Cover, and let marinate in the refrigerator for at least 3 days.

2. Pour the ingredients into a blender, and blend until liquefied.

3. Strain the mixture through a metal sieve or cheesecloth over the jar.

4. Add the vinegar to taste. Shake. This mixture can be used as a simple syrup in homemade sodas, in mocktails, and on ice cream.

Prickly Pear Salad Dressing

Makes 1 cup   **PREP TIME:** *30 minutes*

Prickly pear's flavor is reminiscent of a pineapple, but it also has notes that resemble ripe strawberries, making it a beautiful addition to smoothies, syrups, and salads. Prickly pears are a source of soluble fiber, which can improve gut health and reduce digestive issues like constipation and diarrhea and could also support blood-sugar balance. These tart fruits are a source of antioxidants and vitamin C, which support the immune system, improve skin health, and reduce oxidative stress from physical activity. Prickly pear pulp can also restore important minerals like calcium, magnesium, and potassium to the body; these essential minerals serve as electrolytes and are needed for many functions, including bone, heart, nerve, and muscle health. The electrolytes found in prickly pear fruit can also lessen the effects of a hangover. To consume as a beverage, blend only the first three ingredients and pour over ice with sparkling water.

INGREDIENTS

3 or 4 prickly pear fruit, cut into chunks
3 limes
½ teaspoon sugar
⅓ cup grapeseed oil
¼ teaspoon cayenne
½ teaspoon salt

SUPPLIES

Blender
Metal sieve
Storage container

INSTRUCTIONS

1. Put the prickly pear chunks in a blender, and puree. Strain into an open container.

2. In the blender, combine a minimum of ½ cup of prickly pear puree with the limes, sugar, grapeseed oil, cayenne, and salt. Blend well until the oil is emulsified. Adjust seasonings to taste. Store in the refrigerator, and use within 5 to 7 days.

Red Clover Tea

Makes 2 cups   **PREP TIME:** *25 minutes*

Red clover is a member of the pea family and is commonly used as a ground cover to add nitrogen back to the soil on farmlands. Native to Africa, central Asia, and most of Europe, it is believed red clover was brought to North America around 100 years ago. Native Americans learned how it was used, adopting the plant into their herbal repertoires.

Red clover is considered an "alterative" herb with expectorant qualities. Alterative herbs aid the body in moving out metabolic waste and are thought to purify the blood. This action can have a positive impact on the skin and the immune system. Expectorants work by way of the respiratory system, relieving inflamed lung and bronchial tissue.

Nutritionally, red clover is a source of phytoestrogens; vitamin C; B vitamins such as thiamine and niacin; and the minerals calcium, potassium, and phosphorus. Drinking cold or hot red clover tea is especially replenishing after childbirth or endurance training. The Native Americans consumed red clover infusions medicinally for whooping cough (especially in children), as a kidney aid, and to help with asthma. Red clover can also be used externally for acne, burns, boils, eczema, and vaginal irritation.

INGREDIENTS

6 red clover blossoms
2 cups boiling water
Metal sieve

INSTRUCTIONS

1. Steep the red clover blossoms in the boiling water for at least 20 minutes or up to overnight.

2. Strain out the solids, and enjoy hot or cold.

Lady's Slipper Root Decoction

Makes 1 cup   **PREP TIME:** *5 minutes* / **COOK TIME:** *25 minutes*

Lady's slipper is a medicinal plant native to most of the North American continent and can be found in woodlands and meadows. This flowering plant is also called moccasin flower, both names referring to the shoe-shaped flowers that bloom from May to July; the medicinal roots can be harvested from August to September. A decoction of lady's slipper root is known for its strong sedative effects and ability to reduce spasms. Lady's slipper root was traditionally used to help treat hysteria, epilepsy, nervous headaches, menstrual pain, and insomnia. The Chippewa of the Great Lakes created poultices with the root to calm inflamed skin, applied the powdered root to toothaches, and took small doses for stomach pain.

Due to the strength of lady's slipper root, any preparation should be taken with caution. A water decoction can be taken 1 to 2 tablespoons at a time until your threshold is evaluated. It is noted that some constituents of this root are not extracted in just water, so a tincture preparation may be preferred. Refer to the Cotton-Root Bark Tincture (page 120) recipe for instructions on how to make a lady's slipper root tincture.

INGREDIENTS

1 teaspoon dried lady's
   slipper root
1 cup water

SUPPLIES

Small saucepan
Fine-mesh sieve

INSTRUCTIONS

1. In a small saucepan, combine the root and water. Bring to a boil over medium-high heat. Cook for 3 minutes. Remove from the heat. Cover the pan, and let infuse for 20 minutes.

2. Strain out the solids. Consume in lesser amounts until you achieve the desired effects.

Serenity Cider

Makes 1 cup   **PREP TIME:** *5 minutes* / **COOK TIME:** *5 minutes*

The medicinal action of both California poppy and hops in this delicious cider have sedative and pain-relieving properties. The Cherokee's use of California poppy to "tranquilize the system" is on par with how it is used today. Generally, it is used to quell pain that interrupts sleep and to lessen the feeling of agitation in the nervous system.

Hops are best known for the distinct flavor they add to beers, but Native Americans also discovered their sedative and pain-reducing benefits, using them for toothaches and intestinal pain. Hops belong to the same botanical family as cannabis, the Cannabaceae family. They are both terpene-rich plants that have similar benefits; however, hops do not share the presence of cannabinoids with cannabis. Terpenes are the essential oils of the plant that aid in various physical and mental ailments. Humulene is the main terpene found in hops, and it is noted for its anti-inflammatory properties. The cinnamon stick may seem like just a delicious flavor adornment, but this aromatic herb also supports health by lessening inflammation and balancing blood pressure and blood sugar.

INGREDIENTS

1 cup cranberry juice
1 teaspoon dried
  California poppy
1 teaspoon dried hops
2 whole cloves
1 cinnamon stick
Orange zest or
  peel (optional)

SUPPLIES

Small saucepan
Fine-mesh sieve

INSTRUCTIONS

1. In a small saucepan, combine the cranberry juice, poppy, hops, cloves, cinnamon stick, and orange zest (if using). Bring to a simmer over medium heat. Cook for 5 minutes. Remove from the heat.

2. Strain the mixture, but add the cinnamon stick back to your hot beverage. Enjoy, and invite the slumber!

Sleepy-Time Tincture

Makes 2 cups   **PREP TIME:** *25 minutes, plus at least 4 weeks to infuse*

A lack of sleep can lead to elevated levels of inflammation, blood-sugar imbalances, and mood disorders. Getting enough sleep seems to be one of the easiest things we can do for our health, but statistics show that one in three adults don't get enough sleep. This tincture is best created with fresh milky oats at their peak harvesting time when the "milk" is present, but if this is not possible, dried milky oats are sufficient and supply the body with B vitamins that comfort the nervous system. Valerian is the most common sedative herb suggested by herbalists, and research has found that valerian root can likely improve sleep and reduce anxiety in many people. Albizzia flowers, although not native to North America, currently grow abundantly on the continent and are added to this tincture to decrease insomnia and anxiety.

INGREDIENTS

¼ cup dried or fresh milky oats

¼ cup dried valerian

¼ cup dried albizzia flowers

¼ cup dried chamomile

2 cups 80-proof alcohol

SUPPLIES

4-cup glass jar

Metal sieve

Storage container

Funnel

Dropper bottles

INSTRUCTIONS

1. Put the milky oats, valerian, albizzia flowers, and chamomile in a 4-cup glass jar.

2. Add enough alcohol to cover by 1 inch. Seal the jar tightly, and label. Put in a cool, shady spot, and gently shake every few days for 4 to 6 weeks.

3. To strain, place a sieve over an open container, and pour in the tincture extract. Gently press the plant material to release all fluid.

4. Using a funnel, pour the fluid into dropper bottles. Store in a cool, shady spot for up to 3 years.

Lactation-Support Tea

Makes 2 cups   **PREP TIME:** *10 minutes*

This combination of herbs helps support mothers who are struggling to produce enough milk after childbirth. Red raspberry leaves are astringent and stimulating; the astringency is helpful in toning tissues, making them useful in constricting the uterus after childbirth. In addition, the stimulating aspect aids in the production of breast milk. Oat straw is a source of vitamins, especially B vitamins and minerals that are restorative, allowing for better nutrient uptake and increasing milk flow. Goat's rue is considered a galactagogue, or a medicinal plant that supports lactation, sometimes even in cases where milk has not been produced for an extended period. Goat's rue differs from other herbs because it increases the hormone responsible for producing milk called prolactin, and it has a plant estrogen called genistein, which studies show increases milk storage and the size of the breast tissue. Fenugreek seeds may stimulate mammary glands; however, scientific evidence to confirm this is lacking. Regardless, their flavor is reminiscent of maple syrup, which may entice a baby to latch.

INGREDIENTS

½ cup dried red
   raspberry leaves
½ cup dried oat straw
¼ cup goat's rue
¼ fenugreek seeds

SUPPLIES

Medium mixing bowl
Gloves, for blending
   (optional)
Storage container
4-cup glass jar
Fine-mesh sieve

INSTRUCTIONS

1. To make the tea blend, in a medium bowl, combine the raspberry leaves, oat straw, goat's rue, and fenugreek seeds. Stir to blend well. Transfer to a clean, airtight container. Dried herbal teas retain potency for up to 1 year if stored correctly.

2. To make the tea, put ¼ cup of the herbal tea blend in a 4-cup glass jar, and cover completely with boiling water. Cover loosely with a lid, and let infuse for 10 to 15 minutes.

3. Pour the mixture through a sieve into mugs, and drink hot or cold.

Lovers' Cacao Liqueur

Makes 4 cups

PREP TIME: *10 minutes, plus at least 5 days to infuse /* **COOK TIME:** *30 minutes*

The Menominee considered ginseng to be "the strengthener of mental powers," and the Pawnee called it a "love charm." Considered a reproductive aid for women and men, this root has long been known for its ability to improve stamina in and out of the bedroom.

The Ojibwe way of sustainably harvesting ginseng root, documented in 1932, stated that once the red ginseng berries were mature but had not fallen from the plant, they would harvest the root and plant the berries in the open soil, covering them firmly with soil. They would not return to the location again for three to five years, the amount of time it takes to regrow ginseng root. The commercialization of American ginseng has left this root vulnerable to overharvesting, so if you cannot harvest or buy ethically, consider buying cultivated ginseng root.

FOR THE CHOCOLATE SYRUP

1 cup sugar
1 cup water
½ cup cacao powder

FOR THE CACAO LIQUEUR

10 inches ginseng root
1 tablespoon crushed cardamom pods
1 cinnamon stick
Zest of 3 oranges
3 cups gin or vodka
1 cup homemade chocolate syrup

TO MAKE THE CHOCOLATE SYRUP

1. In a medium saucepan, combine the sugar, water, and cacao powder. Bring to a boil over medium heat. Let slowly boil until reduced by half, or enough to have a viscosity. Remove from the heat. Let cool.

TO MAKE THE CACAO LIQUEUR

2. In a 4-cup widemouthed glass jar, combine the ginseng, cardamom pods, cinnamon stick, and orange zest.

3. Add the gin to cover. Seal the jar, shake to moisten, and store in a cool, dark spot for 5 to 7 days, or until fully infused.

SUPPLIES

Medium saucepan
**4-cup widemouthed
  glass jar**
Metal sieve or strainer
Storage container

4. Strain the herbs from the vodka mixture over an open container. Pour the liquid back into the jar.

5. Pour in the chocolate syrup, and shake well to combine.

6. Sip 1 ounce as desired!

In-the-Mood Electuary

Makes 1¼ cups   **PREP TIME:** *5 minutes*

Electuaries are sweet and sticky, and the taste and sensation of them can help inspire a mood, but this formulation of herbs kicks up the intimacy spice to 100. The cacao nibs in this formula stimulate the production of serotonin and endorphins. They also contain phenylethylamine and anandamide, two chemicals that elevate the mood; help increase focus; and give feelings of attraction, pleasure, and excitement. Maca, a Peruvian root, causes the consumer to feel more energetic, with a sense of well-being, all of which are thought to be due to its ability to restore proper hormone balance. Sarsaparilla root has substances known as phytosterols, which are like testosterone and may stimulate the activity of sex hormones in the body. Sarsaparilla root also brings blood flow to the reproductive organs and may increase the chances of conception. The name "Shatavari" translates to "she who possesses one hundred husbands." As an aphrodisiac, it's used to increase female libido, balance cervical pH, and alleviate dryness.

INGREDIENTS

- 2 tablespoons ground cacao nibs
- 2 tablespoons powdered maca
- 2 tablespoons powdered sarsaparilla root
- 2 tablespoons powdered shatavari
- 1 cup honey

SUPPLIES

Medium mixing bowl
Spatula
Storage container

INSTRUCTIONS

1. In a medium bowl, combine the cacao nibs, maca, sarsaparilla root, and shatavari. Stir until well blended. Transfer to a clean, airtight container. The blend will retain potency for up to 1 year if stored correctly.

2. To create your electuary, combine the desired amount of powdered herbs and honey in a bowl, and stir well. (Other powdered herbs such as cinnamon or ginger can be added if you want more flavor or need to make the mixture thicker for rolling into balls.) Consume 1 to 2 teaspoons at desired times.

Black Cohosh Tea

Serves 1   **PREP TIME:** *5 minutes* / **COOK TIME:** *25 minutes*

Native Americans used black cohosh to treat a variety of gynecological issues, including PMS and menopausal symptoms. Studies have associated the use of black cohosh with a decreased risk of breast cancer, and evidence supports its use for decreasing fibroid size and treating PCOS symptoms, menstrual disorders, and hot flashes. Some of these results could be due to black cohosh containing phytoestrogens, which mimic estrogens within the female body. Black cohosh may also be recommended by a midwife to induce labor in the third trimester and is not an herb to be consumed earlier in pregnancy. Ginger is also an herb that quells inflammation, decreasing menstrual cramps and reducing the digestive discomfort associated with hormonal fluctuations.

Decocting is the method used to coax out all the active constituents of hard roots and seeds and is best done for at least 30 minutes. However, the resulting brew will be slightly bitter and can be tempered with a sweetener. If you are choosing to steep your root, just be aware it will not have the same medicinal potency as a decoction. Another effective way of taking in the medicinal benefits of black cohosh is through a tincture.

INGREDIENTS

1 teaspoon dried black cohosh root
8 to 12 ounces water
½ teaspoon dried gingerroot
Honey or sugar, for serving

SUPPLIES

Small saucepan
Metal sieve or strainer

INSTRUCTIONS

1. In a small saucepan, combine the black cohosh, water, and ginger. Bring to a boil over medium heat. Cook for 20 to 30 minutes. Remove from the heat. (For a milder brew, steep roots in boiled water for 5 to 10 minutes.)

2. Strain the mixture over a mug, and add honey to taste.

Cotton-Root Bark Tincture

Makes 1 to 1½ cups   **PREP TIME:** *10 minutes, plus at least 4 weeks to infuse*

Cotton-root bark has been traditionally used by midwives to increase uterine contractions at the end of pregnancy, expel the afterbirth, and increase milk production during lactation. It can also be used in the case of irregular menstruation, painful menstrual cramps, and for symptoms associated with menopause. Anecdotal evidence suggests that cotton-root bark can be used as an aphrodisiac.

This recipe uses the "folk" method, with alcohol as the solvent. This method requires little measurement math but still creates an effective solution.

INGREDIENTS

½ cup dried cotton-root
  bark, cut into
  small pieces
1½ cups
  80-proof alcohol

SUPPLIES

Cutting board and knife
Glass jar
Metal sieve
Storage container
Funnel
Dropper bottles

INSTRUCTIONS

1. Put the cotton-root bark in a glass jar, and add enough alcohol to cover by 1 inch. Seal the jar tightly, and label. Put in a cool, dark spot, and shake gently every few days for 4 to 6 weeks.

2. To strain, place a sieve over an open container, and pour in the tincture extract. Gently press the plant material to release all fluid.

3. Using a funnel, pour the fluid into dropper bottles. Tinctures have a long shelf life of 1 to 3 years.

Black Haw and Cramp Bark Relief Decoction

Makes 4 cups **PREP TIME:** *5 minutes* / **COOK TIME:** *20 minutes*

Black haw and cramp bark are two barks that are considered uterine antispasmodics, meaning they relax the smooth muscles of the uterus and can work separately or together to lessen the pain of menstruation, as well as back pain and pain that radiates down the thighs. Taken in either a decoction or tincture, they can be consumed a few days leading up to the menstruation cycle to prevent pain or at the onset of pain. Cramp bark, just like black haw, has been traditionally used to stop premature contractions in early pregnancy that can lead to miscarriage. Using both plants concurrently increases the likelihood of pain relief.

Because both are barks, the method to extract the active constituents is by decoction. When decocting, the plant matter will be boiled for an extended amount of time to break through the cellular wall. These two plants can also be tinctured together at a 1-to-1 ratio; refer to the Cotton-Root Bark Tincture (page 120) recipe for how to create a black haw/cramp bark tincture.

INGREDIENTS

2 tablespoons dried black haw bark

2 tablespoons dried cramp bark

4½ cups water

SUPPLIES

Medium saucepan

Metal sieve

4-cup glass jar with lid

INSTRUCTIONS

1. In a medium saucepan, combine the black haw bark, cramp bark, and water. Bring to a boil over medium-high heat, about 5 to 10 minutes.

2. Reduce the heat to the lowest simmer point. Cover the pan, and simmer for 10 minutes. Remove from the heat.

3. Strain the roots out of decoction over a 4-cup glass jar. Label, and store in the refrigerator for up to 3 days. Consume ½ cup up to three times a day as needed for the prevention or treatment of cramps.

Gotu Kola Tissue-Regeneration Tea

Makes 1 cup   **PREP TIME:** *10 minutes*

Healing tissue throughout the body requires a diet high in minerals and vitamins. It can be challenging to get enough of these vital nutrients through meals alone, especially if the body is undergoing a trauma that alters appetite. Nutritive herbs can fill in nutritional gaps, and the nutrients often have greater bioavailability than multivitamin tablets because they are in a whole-food form. Gotu kola is the primary herb in this tea because it has asiaticoside, which, according to studies, increases collagen production and tissue regeneration, leading to quicker healing of wounds and a reduction in scarring. Vitamin C is also critical for the formation of collagen, and that is sourced from the rose hips, an herb that also offers lubrication to the cells. Spearmint is a source of magnesium, a mineral that promotes the development of stem cells in cartilage. This tea blend is rounded out by the anti-inflammatory herb turmeric, which can be replaced with gingerroot for taste preference; both decrease inflammation and increase circulation.

INGREDIENTS

¼ cup dried gotu kola
¼ cup dried rose hips
¼ cup dried spearmint
¼ cup dried turmeric
8 to 12 ounces
   boiling water

SUPPLIES

Medium mixing bowl
Gloves, for blending
   (optional)
Storage container

INSTRUCTIONS

1. To make the tea blend, in a medium bowl, combine the gotu kola, rose hips, spearmint, and turmeric. Stir until well blended. Transfer to a clean, airtight container. The blend will retain potency for up to 1 year if stored correctly.

2. To make a cup of tea, steep 2 tablespoons of the herbal tea blend in the boiling water for 5 to 10 minutes.

Bone Health Super Infusion

Makes 1 cup   **PREP TIME:** *10 minutes, plus overnight to infuse*

Many of the medicinal plants Native Americans historically consumed served nutritional purposes as well as medicinal ones, supplying the body with the vitamins and minerals to sustain strong muscles and bones. The first of these nutritive herbs in this tea recipe is horsetail, a plant source of the mineral silicon that protects the bones from calcium loss. Alfalfa, a source of vitamin K, positively affects bone density and supports bone repair after breakdown. Manganese is a mineral that also has a role in bone formation and is found in spearmint, the aromatic herb that adds a refreshing flavor to this bone-supporting tea. Last, red clover, a medicinal flower in the pea family brought over with European settlers, has isoflavones that encourage bone-building activity. For menopausal women, the phytoestrogens in red clover mimic estrogen, helping prevent bone loss. Creating this as a super infusion includes larger amounts of herbs than traditional herbal teas and longer infusing times to extract as many nutrients as possible.

INGREDIENTS

¼ cup horsetail
¼ cup alfalfa
¼ cup spearmint
¼ cup red clover

SUPPLIES

Medium mixing bowl
Gloves, for blending
  (optional)
4-cup glass jar with lid
Metal sieve

INSTRUCTIONS

1. To make the tea blend, in a medium bowl, combine the horsetail, alfalfa, spearmint, and red clover. Stir until well blended. Transfer to a clean, airtight container. The blend will retain potency for up to 1 year if stored correctly.

2. To make a super infusion, place ¼ cup of herbs in a 4-cup glass jar. Cover with boiled water, stir, and loosely cap with the lid. Let sit overnight, strain, and drink hot or cold.

Herb-Infused Bone Broth

Makes 6 cups

PREP TIME: *15 minutes /*
COOK TIME: *4 hours 10 minutes*

Creating your own bone broth increases the nutrient density, reduces food waste, and enhances the health of your whole body to include bone health, digestive health, and enhanced immunity. Making your own broth also allows you to get creative with the ingredients you add; for example, the recipe calls for whole vegetables, but instead you can use vegetable scraps from past meals, or you may want to add a larger variety of immune-supportive or mineral-rich herbs. The herbs in the following recipe help repair the gut lining, supporting more efficient nutrient uptake and digestion. The bones and especially chicken feet are a rich source of collagen, complementing the herbs' effects on the lining of the stomach; lubricating the joints; and supporting the growth of healthy hair, skin, and nails. A well-executed bone broth will become gelatinous when chilled and can be warmed and sipped in lieu of tea or added to your favorite recipes.

INGREDIENTS

1 tablespoon olive oil
Mixture of onions,
  carrots, and
  celery, chopped
3 garlic cloves,
  finely chopped
1 gallon water
1 pound chicken bones,
  chicken feet, or both
2 tablespoons apple
  cider vinegar
¼ cup calendula
  flowers
¼ cup dried
  burdock root

INSTRUCTIONS

1. In a large stockpot, heat the oil over medium heat.

2. Add onions, carrots, and celery. Sauté until translucent.

3. Add the garlic, and cook for 2 minutes.

**3 tablespoons
plantain leaves
1 or 2 slices dried reishi
1 tablespoon
seaweed flakes, or
2 strips (optional)**

SUPPLIES

**Large stockpot
Large fine-mesh
strainer
Storage container**

4. Reduce the heat to medium-low. Add the water, chicken components, vinegar, calendula flowers, burdock root, plantain leaves, reishi, and seaweed (if using). Simmer for 4 hours. Remove from the heat.

5. Strain all the ingredients over a container. Your broth can be consumed on its own or used to make a soup. Store in the refrigerator for up to 7 days.

Modern-Day Pemmican

Makes 12 bars   **PREP TIME:** *1 hour*

Traditionally, pemmican is made of tallow, meat, and dried fruits. The dried fruits available would be those that were native to the hunting grounds and would include huckleberries, chokecherries, elderberries, and cranberries. Any meat that was sourced that season could be blended with the other components to create a calorie- and protein-rich food bar or cake that would be stored for use throughout the year. This recipe is a modern twist with an increased nutritional profile from the herbs and nuts. The ingredients can easily be mixed and matched; the main goal is that the consistency is tacky enough to create bars. Regardless of the natural ingredients you use, this compact meal will be plentiful in good fats, nutrient-rich vegetables, herbs, and fiber-rich berries.

INGREDIENTS

¼ cup coconut oil

1 cup dried meat
  or jerky

¼ cup ground walnuts

¼ cup dried
  nettle leaves

¼ cup dried cherries

¼ cup dried blueberries

¼ cup dried prunes

2 dried figs

SUPPLIES

Microwave-safe bowl
Microwave
Food processor
Spatula
8 x 8-inch baking dish

INSTRUCTIONS

1. Put the coconut oil in a microwave-safe bowl, and microwave on high until the oil has melted.

2. In a food processor, combine the meat, walnuts, nettle leaves, cherries, blueberries, prunes, figs, and warmed coconut oil. Blend until fully incorporated.

3. Using a spatula, remove the mixture and transfer to an 8 x 8-inch baking or storage dish. Press down until ¾ inch thick. Make sure all the air bubbles are out.

4. Chill the mixture until firm. If you prefer bars, cut the mixture into bars after chilling for a few hours. Store in the refrigerator for up to 10 days.

Pineapple Weed and Coconut Granola

Makes 5 cups **PREP TIME:** *25 minutes* / **COOK TIME:** *20 minutes*

Also known as wild chamomile or disc mayweed, pineapple weed is a low-growing weed that grows in sunny gravel lots and protrudes out between sidewalk cracks. Pineapple weed has a bright yellow button or disc body that, when crushed, exudes the scent of pineapple and tastes similar to it. Medicinal uses of pineapple weed mirror that of chamomile, such as alleviating tummy woes and pain and promoting relaxation. The delicious flavor and the antioxidant benefits of this wild plant lead to its use in unique and nutritious recipes.

INGREDIENTS

- ¼ cup fresh or dried pineapple weed
- ½ cup maple syrup
- ½ cup coconut oil
- ½ teaspoon ground cinnamon
- ½ teaspoon salt
- 3 cups rolled oats
- ½ cup dried coconut
- ½ cup dried pineapple

SUPPLIES

- Small mixing bowl
- Spatula
- Baking sheet
- Parchment paper
- Large mixing bowl
- Storage container

INSTRUCTIONS

1. In a small bowl, combine the pineapple weed, maple syrup, coconut oil, cinnamon, and salt. Stir until well blended. Set aside to fully infuse while completing the next steps.

2. Preheat the oven to 300°F. Line a baking sheet with parchment paper.

3. In a large bowl, combine the oats, dried coconut, and dried pineapple. Mix well.

4. Pour the wet ingredients into the dry ingredients, and mix until fully combined.

5. Spread the mixture evenly onto the prepared baking sheet.

6. Transfer the baking sheet to the oven, and bake, stirring at least once, for 20 minutes, or until the granola is golden brown. Remove from the oven. Let cool completely before transferring to a clean, airtight container. Store in a cabinet or pantry for up to 1 month.

Sumac Lemonade

Makes 2 cups   **PREP TIME:** *4 hours*

If you are lucky enough to come across sumac that is ripe and ready for harvest, you can dry it to blend and use as a lemony-earthy-flavored spice to make a tangy and refreshing beverage later or use immediately for this recipe. The most difficult aspect of this recipe is harvesting the sumac and waiting the extended amount of time for the berries to infuse the water enough for you to fully enjoy. Sumac lemonade is a fun way to introduce plants and their benefits to children and new wildcrafters. This refreshing drink will fill your cells with antioxidants that reduce inflammation and support heart health and healthy blood sugar.

INGREDIENTS

2 clusters fresh
   sumac berries
4 cups cool or
   room-temperature
   water, divided
Your preferred
   sweetener, for serving

SUPPLIES

4-cup glass jar
Muddler or similar tool
Storage container

INSTRUCTIONS

1. Put the berries in a 4-cup glass jar, and add 1 cup of water.

2. Using a muddler, crush the berries.

3. Add the remaining water. Let the sumac berries infuse the water for at least 3 to 4 hours. The longer the period of time, the more intense the flavor will be.

4. Strain the pulp over an open container, and return the liquid to the jar.

5. Sweeten with your preferred sweetener, and enjoy.

Ultimate Tonic Tea

Makes 2 cups   **PREP TIME:** *20 minutes*

Nutritive herbs are rich in vitamins and minerals; they supply a source of easily assimilated nutrients. Many overlook the valuable nutritional aspect of herbs in favor of what they offer during acute health challenges, but herbs have always served as a nutritive food source for Native Americans, supplying the building blocks to a body that can withstand the many challenges of life. Nettles, oat straw, and red raspberry leaves are all sources of minerals, including chromium, iron, calcium, potassium, magnesium, manganese, silica, and phosphorus. When combined with the rose hips in this tea, you'll receive vitamins A, C, D, E, K, and myriad B vitamins.

This tea recipe is fully customizable, and you can add and subtract herbs to your liking. Eleuthero is added as an adaptogen to restore stamina and to boost the body's resistance to stress, but it can also be swapped out for another adaptogen, such as reishi mushroom, ashwagandha, or astragalus.

INGREDIENTS

½ cup nettle leaves
½ cup oat straw
½ cup red
  raspberry leaves
¼ cup eleuthero root
¼ cup rose hips
8 to 12 ounces
  boiling water

SUPPLIES

Medium mixing bowl
Gloves, for blending
  (optional)
Storage container

INSTRUCTIONS

1. To make the tea blend, in a medium mixing bowl, combine the nettle leaves, oat straw, raspberry leaves, eleuthero root, and rose hips. Stir until well blended. Transfer to a clean, airtight container. The blend will retain potency for up to 1 year if stored correctly.

2. To make a cup of tea, steep 2 teaspoons of the herbal tea blend in the boiling water for 10 to 20 minutes.

Mountain Mint Mouthwash

Makes 4 cups   **PREP TIME:** *15 minutes*

Mountain mint is an important pollinator plant, with several species growing throughout North America, blooming in late summer to early fall depending on where you are finding the plant. This mint is more mentholated than other mints and gives a cooling sensation. The Lakota used this aromatic mint to quell coughs, and the Cherokee created an infusion with it including green corn to prevent diarrhea. Currently, mountain mint is recognized for its help in healing gum disease, mouth sores, and tooth pain. Due to its analgesic and antiseptic properties, this medicinal herb is ideal for mouthwash. Parsley, like many plants, has bacteria-fighting chlorophyll, which is the chemical that gives the herb its dark green color. Adding the vodka and orange essential oil will increase the shelf life for this mouthwash, and for extra reassurance, you can store it in the refrigerator.

INGREDIENTS

2 cups water
¼ cup dried
   mountain mint
2 tablespoons
   dried parsley
2 tablespoons vodka
4 drops orange
   essential oil (optional)

SUPPLIES

Medium saucepan
Infuser or metal sieve
Glass jar

INSTRUCTIONS

1. In a medium saucepan, bring the water to a boil over medium-high heat.

2. Add the mountain mint and parsley in a fillable tea bag, in an infuser, or loose. Remove from the heat. Let steep for 10 minutes.

3. Strain the mixture over a glass jar, or remove the tea bag or infuser and pour into a jar.

4. Once cool, add the vodka (as a preservative), and essential oil (if using).

5. To use: Swish ½ to 1 ounce mouthwash as needed.

Antibacterial Healing Herb Liniment

Makes 1 cup   **PREP TIME:** *20 minutes, plus 4 weeks to infuse*

A liniment is an external application of herbal medicines used for drying, drawing, and disinfecting or for relief of deep muscle pain. Liniments are created similarly to tinctures; however, the solvent extracting the medicinal components of the herbs is rubbing alcohol. This liniment can be used as a disinfectant for weeping infections, including boils, pimples, and poison oak or ivy. Additionally, it can be used on athlete's foot. When safely stored in a cool, dark spot, liniments will keep almost indefinitely.

The prominent Native American herb in this formula is goldenseal. This medicinal root has been historically valued for its antibacterial, antimicrobial, and anti-inflammatory properties and was used by the Cherokee and Haudenosaunee to medicate the ears and eyes. Goldenseal root has experienced overharvesting for commercialization and has been placed on the United Plant Savers' "at-risk" list, so be sure your product is ethically sourced. Goldenseal is a berberine-rich plant like goldthread, which is also overharvested, but both can be replaced with Oregon grape root.

INGREDIENTS

1 ounce powdered goldenseal root

1 ounce dried comfrey

1 ounce dried calendula flowers

1 pint rubbing alcohol

SUPPLIES

Widemouthed jar

Metal sieve

Cheesecloth

Storage container

INSTRUCTIONS

1. Put the goldenseal root, comfrey, and calendula flowers in a widemouthed jar.

2. Pour in the rubbing alcohol to cover by 2 inches. Seal the jar, and label. Store in a cool, shady spot. Shake the jar every 1 to 3 days for 4 weeks.

3. After 4 weeks, strain the mixture over a new container. A spray bottle is best.

Baby Balm

Makes 1 cup   **PREP TIME:** *5 minutes* / **COOK TIME:** *45 minutes*

Calendula is a cultivated herb known for its first aid benefit. Traveling to the North American continent with European settlers, calendula was used during the Civil War to stop bleeding and heal wounds. This balm can be used on burns, bruises, and scrapes. It can be used to treat muscle spasms. And it can even be used on baby bottoms. It has antibacterial and anti-inflammatory properties and is a source of wrinkle-reducing vitamins A and C.

INGREDIENTS

¼ cup dried
   calendula flowers
2 tablespoons
   dried lavender
1 cup coconut oil or
   olive oil
½ cup dried herbs
1 ounce beeswax
   pellets

SUPPLIES

Double boiler
Metal sieve
Cheesecloth
Storage containers

INSTRUCTIONS

1. Place the calendula, lavender, coconut oil, and dried herbs in the top of a double boiler.

2. Bring water in the bottom of the double boiler to a slow boil over medium heat. Let the herbs and oils infuse for 30 minutes to 1 hour.

3. Once the herbs have completely infused your oil, using a sieve and cheesecloth, strain the mixture over a container. Make sure to squeeze the excess oil from your spent herbs, and compost them. Return the oil to the top of the double boiler.

4. Add the beeswax, and warm over low heat until the oil and wax have fully emulsified. Remove from the heat. You can check your mixture for solidity by putting a spoonful on a plate and chilling it in the freezer for 5 to 10 minutes. If the mixture is too soft for your liking, add more beeswax 1 teaspoon at a time.

5. Pour the salve into containers while hot and allow to solidify before sealing to avoid condensation. Salve expiration times vary from 3 months to 1 year; it depends on the volatility of the oils and amount of beeswax. Look for signs of aging, such as separation, mold, or an off-putting smell.

Burdock and Rosemary Skin and Hair Rinse

Makes 2 cups   **PREP TIME:** *10 minutes* / **COOK TIME:** *20 minutes*

Burdock is a root that not only is nutritional and medicinal internally but also has external benefits for the skin and hair. Native Americans historically used burdock washes for swelling and sores that would ooze, implicating that it would be an external treatment for acne sores. Internally, it purifies the blood, ridding the body of excess hormones that could be a culprit in excessive outbreaks. Horsetail was used for myriad purposes among the Native Americans, including lowering high blood pressure, supporting kidney health, and addressing gynecological and dermatological concerns. Today, we know that horsetail is a source of silica, a nutrient that enhances the health and growth of the skin, hair, and nails.

Rosemary is a shrub native to the Mediterranean that has a stimulating effect, encouraging hair growth. Peppermint and lavender are two herbs that can be added for similar effects.

INGREDIENTS

1 cup fresh burdock root, peeled and diced, or ½ cup dried burdock

2 cups water

3 rosemary sprigs, or 1 tablespoon dried rosemary

2 tablespoons dried horsetail

SUPPLIES

Small saucepan
Metal sieve
Storage containers

INSTRUCTIONS

1. In a small saucepan, combine the burdock, water, rosemary, and horsetail. Bring to a boil over medium-high heat, about 5 to 10 minutes.

2. Reduce the heat to medium-low. Simmer for 15 minutes. Remove from the heat.

3. Strain the mixture over a storage container. (Storage options include a spray bottle, narrow toner bottle, or jar.) Let cool. Store in the refrigerator for up to 10 days.

4. To use: Spray in hair or on face, use a cotton pad to swipe over skin, or pour over hair in the bath.

Jewelweed Salve

Makes 1 cup   **PREP TIME:** *5 minutes* / **COOK TIME:** *45 minutes*

Jewelweed is a medicinal plant that has historically been used by the Cherokee, Haudenosaunee, and others to treat the effects of poison ivy, hives for babies, and the stinging from nettle leaves. This salve recipe serves in the same way as an herbal infusion, treating a variety of topical ailments such as bugbites, eczema, itchy skin, psoriasis, and wind-chapped skin.

INGREDIENTS

**1 cup coconut oil or
   olive oil**
¼ cup dried jewelweed
**1 ounce
   beeswax pellets**

SUPPLIES

Double boiler
Metal sieve
Cheesecloth
Storage containers

INSTRUCTIONS

1. Place the oil and dried jewelweed in the top of a double boiler.

2. Bring water in the bottom of the double boiler to a slow boil over medium heat. Let the herbs and oils infuse for 30 minutes to 1 hour.

3. Once the herbs have completely infused the oil, using a sieve and cheesecloth, strain the mixture over a container. Make sure to squeeze the excess oil from your spent herbs and compost them. Return the oil to the top of the double boiler.

4. Add the beeswax, and warm over low heat until the oil and wax have fully emulsified. Remove from the heat. You can check your mixture for solidity by putting a spoonful on a plate and putting it in the freezer for 5 to 10 minutes. If the mixture is too soft for your liking, add more beeswax 1 teaspoon at a time.

5. Pour the salve into containers while hot, and let solidify before sealing to avoid condensation. Salve expiration times vary from 3 months to 1 year, depending on the volatility of the oils and the amount of beeswax. Look for signs of aging, such as separation, mold, or an off-putting smell.

Plantain Salve

Makes 1 cup   **PREP TIME:** *5 minutes* / **COOK TIME:** *45 minutes*

Plantain leaf was also known as the Englishman's foot because it came over with colonists and was believed to grow in every area the settlers stepped foot. Plantain leaves have polysaccharides that promote the repair of skin tissue. They are moisturizing and possess anti-inflammatory properties. This salve is ideal for inclusion in your first aid kit to heal minor skin abrasions, insect stings, and burns.

INGREDIENTS

¼ cup dried
   plantain leaves
1 cup coconut oil or
   olive oil
1 ounce
   beeswax pellets
½ cup dried herbs

SUPPLIES

Double boiler
Metal sieve
Cheesecloth
Storage containers

INSTRUCTIONS

1. Place the dried plantain leaves and oil in the top of a double boiler.

2. Bring water in the bottom of the double boiler to a slow boil over medium heat. Let the herbs and oils infuse for 30 minutes to 1 hour.

3. Once the herbs have completely infused the oil, using a sieve and cheesecloth, strain the mixture over a container. Make sure to squeeze the excess oil from your spent herbs and compost them. Return the oil to the top of the double boiler.

4. Add the beeswax, and warm over low heat until the oil and wax have fully emulsified. Remove from the heat. You can check your mixture for solidity by putting a spoonful on a plate and putting it in the freezer for 5 to 10 minutes. If the mixture is too soft for your liking, add more beeswax 1 teaspoon at a time.

5. Pour the salve into containers while hot, and let solidify before sealing to avoid condensation. Salve expiration times vary from 3 months to 1 year, depending on the volatility of the oils and the amount of beeswax. Look for signs of aging, such as separation, mold, or an off-putting smell.

Pennyroyal Pest Spray

Makes 2 cups   **PREP TIME:** *25 minutes*

Pennyroyal is a member of the mint family and grows throughout North America. This aromatic, low-growing herb can be found in open woodlands and in flat hills with sun exposure. It has a square stem and leaves that are arranged opposite of one another, ovate-shaped, and about a half an inch long. Pennyroyal spreads through underground vines and blooms small purple flowers from late winter to spring.

Among many other uses, Native American tribes consumed pennyroyal infusions as contraception and as an abortifacient, or abortion-inducing herb. Due to this ability to stimulate the uterus, it can also be used to promote menstruation; however, this action makes pennyroyal an herb to use internally with caution. Externally, pennyroyal can be used as an insect repellent to deter chiggers, fleas, and mosquitoes. Because pennyroyal can be harmful to domesticated animals such as cats and dogs, this spray should not be used around pets. These plants can also be used in essential-oil form.

INGREDIENTS

1 cup water

1 tablespoon dried pennyroyal

1 tablespoon dried peppermint

½ tablespoon dried lavender

1 cup witch hazel

SUPPLIES

Small saucepan

Metal sieve

Funnel

Storage container (a glass spray bottle is ideal)

INSTRUCTIONS

1. In a small saucepan, bring the water to a boil over medium-high heat. Remove from the heat.

2. Add the pennyroyal, peppermint, and lavender. Cover the pan, and let infuse for 10 minutes.

3. Once cooled, add the witch hazel. Strain the mixture over a container. Be sure to label as "for external use only." Store for up to 6 months.

Yucca Root Liquid Soap

Makes 2 cups

PREP TIME: *10 minutes, plus at least 4 hours to infuse /*
COOK TIME: *1 hour 45 minutes*

Yucca, also known as soapweed, has been traditionally used among many tribes, including the Cheyenne, Navajo, and Kiowa Tribes, for dermatological purposes. It is used to treat inflamed dry skin, dandruff, hair loss, and lice. Yucca has natural saponins, which lather in the presence of water, so it can be used as a cleansing agent while offering emollient or moisturizing benefits.

INGREDIENTS

3½ ounces yucca root, cut into 1-inch dice

2 cups distilled water, divided

2 tablespoons dried sage

2 tablespoons vegetable glycerin

Essential oils of your preference (optional)

SUPPLIES

Digital scale

Cutting board and sharp knife

Food processor

Baking sheet

Parchment paper

Small saucepan

Storage container

INSTRUCTIONS

1. Put the yucca in a food processor, and pulverize into smaller pieces.

2. Preheat the oven to 200°F. Line a baking sheet with parchment paper.

3. Spread the yucca evenly over the prepared baking sheet.

4. Transfer the baking sheet to the oven, and bake for at least 1 hour, or until completely dried. Remove from the oven.

5. Put ¼ cup of distilled water and the sage in a jar. Let infuse for 4 to 6 hours.

6. In a small saucepan, combine the dried yucca root with the remaining distilled water. Bring to a boil over medium-high heat. Cook for 10 minutes.

7. Reduce the heat to a simmer. Cook until the root has completely dissolved. The mixture will be frothy. Watch to avoid boiling over. Remove from the heat.

8. Combine the yucca mixture with the sage infusion, and add the vegetable glycerin. Stir to combine.

9. Cool the mixture, and pour into a storage container. Your homemade liquid soap will stay fresh for up to 2 months.

Wild Rice Skin Exfoliator

Makes 6 tablespoons   **PREP TIME:** *10 minutes*

Wild rice has been an important cultural food for the Ojibwe people of the Great Lakes for more than twelve thousand years. The story that is passed down through generations says that there were eight prophets that delivered seven prophecies for them to follow, and the third prophecy was to go west until they found land where food grew on water. Their western migration ended when they found beds of wild rice growing in the Great Lakes region. This is where they settled, and through perseverance and initiative, they continue to grow wild rice in a way that honors their ancestors. Traditional harvesting of this rice is done from the end of August to mid-September, during the "wild rice–making moon," with only motorless canoes allowed in the rice paddies.

Rice powders have been used in Asia for centuries to calm inflammation and cleanse impurities from pores. Also, the chemical structure of rice is like the ceramides in the skin, encouraging the production of collagen.

INGREDIENTS

6 tablespoons wild rice
¼ cup water

SUPPLIES

Food processor
  or blender
Storage container
Small mixing bowl
Stirring spatula

INSTRUCTIONS

1. To make the rice flour, in a food processor or blender, blend the preferred amount of rice until finely ground. Store in a clean, airtight container for up to 1 year.

2. When ready to use, in a small bowl, mix 2 tablespoons of the rice flour with the water to create a paste. Using a circular motion, smooth over your face. Allow the mask to sit for 10 minutes before removing.

Licorice Root Throat Spray

Makes ½ cup   **PREP TIME:** *25 minutes, plus 2 weeks to infuse*

Licorice root grows natively throughout Canada, every western and midwestern state, and some upper eastern states. This sweet, moisturizing root was chewed by tribal members to strengthen their throats for singing or to heal a sore throat. The Cheyenne people of the Great Plains knew it as a digestive herb that could halt diarrhea, and the Lakota chewed licorice root for tooth pain.

Licorice root has anti-inflammatory, antimicrobial, and antioxidant properties, and its sweetness comes from the constituent glycyrrhizin. This sweetness, along with the moisturizing qualities, offers a soothing sensation to bronchial and digestive tissues and is recommended in the presence of dry coughs or throats. Be aware, however, some consumers may experience negative side effects of hypertension and irregular heartbeat from the glycyrrhizin present in licorice root, so it is best to use with caution in smaller amounts for short periods of time.

INGREDIENTS

3 tablespoons dried
  licorice root
¼ cup water
3 tablespoons honey
¼ cup vodka

SUPPLIES

2-cup glass jar
Small saucepan
Small metal sieve
Funnel
Spray bottles

INSTRUCTIONS

1. Put the licorice root in a 2-cup glass jar.

2. In a small saucepan, bring the water to a boil over medium-high heat. Remove from the heat. Pour over the licorice root.

3. Add the honey, cover the jar, and let steep for 15 minutes.

4. Add the vodka, and stir well to combine. Seal the jar, put in a dark spot, and let infuse for 2 weeks.

5. Strain the herbs from the tincture, and funnel the tincture into spray bottles. Use within 3 months.

6. To use, spray directly into the back of the affected throat.

Urinary Tract Support Tea

Makes 1 cup   **PREP TIME:** *10 minutes*

"Pipsissewa," from traditional Cree language, means "to break into small pieces," and is in reference to this medicinal herb's ability to break kidney stones into small pieces so they can be more easily expelled from the body. Pipsissewa is also a diuretic, stimulating urine flow, and an antiseptic working primarily in the urinary and reproductive systems. Topically, pipsissewa's antiseptic properties can heal blisters, stings, sores, and scratches. Documented use of this native herb included several tribes throughout North America, from the Salish Tribes on the West Coast to the Abenaki peoples of the northeast woodlands of Canada and south to the Catawba Tribe of South Carolina that referred to pipsissewa as "fire flower" and knew of its analgesic properties for back pain.

Uva ursi is equally as supportive to the urinary system as pipsissewa. A compound present in this herb called arbutin converts to hydroquinone, a substance that is antimicrobial. Pipsissewa is considered safe for most individuals; however, uva ursi is not recommended for children or those who are pregnant or nursing.

INGREDIENTS

8 to 12 ounces water
1 teaspoon dried
  pipsissewa leaves
1 teaspoon dried uva
  ursi leaves

SUPPLIES

Kettle or
  small saucepan
Infuser, fillable tea
  bags, or strainer
  and container
Hot-beverage mug

INSTRUCTIONS

1. In a kettle or small saucepan, bring the water to a boil over medium-high heat. Remove from the heat.

2. Put the pipsissewa and uva ursi into an infuser or fillable tea bags, and place in a hot-beverage mug. Or, if using a strainer, put the herbs in an open container.

3. Pour the hot water over the herbs, and let steep for 10 to 15 minutes.

4. Remove the infuser or tea bags, or pour the mixture through the strainer into a mug to remove the herbs. Drink 2 to 3 cups a day to relieve symptoms.

Water-Release Tea

Makes desired amount   **PREP TIME:** *10 minutes*

This blend of herbs helps release water weight, acts as a cleanser to the urinary tract, and eases digestion. The peppermint lifts this blend of urinary-supporting herbs and offers a mild mint flavor to balance the astringency of the other herbs. Dandelion leaf releases excess water weight, nettles are an herbal diuretic and restore vital minerals such as potassium and magnesium, and corn silk flushes the kidneys of toxins.

Blending loose-leaf herbal teas is one of the simplest of herbal preparations. I prefer to measure in parts; for example, 1 teaspoon can equal 1 part, or ¼ cup can equal 1 part. Parts can be teaspoons, tablespoons, or ⅛-cup to 1-cup units, creating the batch size you desire. The part size you choose will be based on how much tea you would like to make. Adding dried fruit to any tea blend can increase the health benefits and the natural sweetness.

INGREDIENTS

3 parts dried peppermint leaves

2 parts dried nettle leaves

1 part dried dandelion leaves

½ part dried corn silk

Sprinkle of dried chopped cranberries (optional)

8 to 12 ounces boiling water

SUPPLIES

Medium mixing bowl

Gloves, for blending (optional)

Storage container

INSTRUCTIONS

1. To make the tea blend, in a medium bowl, combine the peppermint, nettle, dandelion, corn silk, and cranberries (if using). Stir until well blended. Transfer to a clean, airtight container. The blend will retain potency for up to 1 year if stored correctly.

2. To make a cup of tea, steep 2 teaspoons of the herbal tea blend in the boiling water for 5 to 10 minutes.

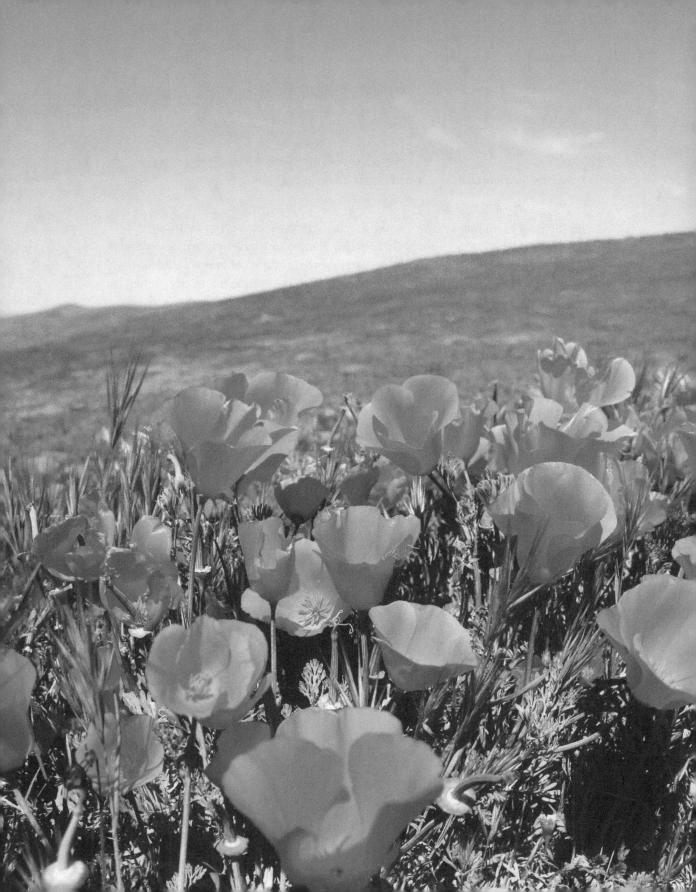

RESOURCES

Books

Braiding Sweetgrass by Robin Wall Kimmerer. A book of stories and Indigenous wisdom that invites us to take notice of the natural world.

The Medicine Wheel Garden by herbalist and ethnobotanist E. Barrie Kavasch. This book is a guide to planting herbs in the style of a medicine wheel.

Native Plant Stories by Joseph Bruchac. For adults and children, this book is a collection of short mythological stories about plants from eighteen different Native American tribes.

Plants Have So Much to Give Us, All We Have to Do Is Ask by Mary Siisip Geniusz. This book emulates how Native Americans used storytelling to teach about medicinal plants.

Restoring the Kinship Worldview by Wahinkpe Topa and Darcia Narvaez. Perspectives from Indigenous leaders on how to come back into balance with life on earth.

The World We Used to Live In by Vine Deloria Jr. This book is an examination of Native American spirituality before modern commercialization.

Websites

American Herbalists Guild | An association of herbal practitioners (AmericanHerbalistsGuild.com): Learn how to become a registered herbalist and to locate a professional herbalist that has met the educational guidelines of the group.

California Native Plant Society (CNPS) (CNPS.org): A nonprofit dedicated to conserving California's native plants and their habitats, including educational resources on the appropriation of white sage.

Children's Dosage Guide | Herb lore (HerbLore.com/overviews/childrens
-dosage-guide): This site offers a breakdown of the three "rules" discussed in
chapter 1, "Be Mindful of Herbal Dosage."

Henriette's Herbal Homepage (Henriettes-Herb.com): One of the oldest herbal
resources on the internet, offers extensive resources on each herb.

Native Circle | Native American history and culture, Indian words of wisdom,
politics, and arts (NativeCircle.com): An easy-to-navigate educational website that
touches on Native American spirituality, history, and art.

Native-Land.ca | Our home on Native land (Native-Land.ca): Enter your zip code
on the site to learn who the First Peoples were to inhabit the land on which you
currently reside.

REFERENCES

Anderson, Kat M. "The Original Medicinal Plant Gatherers & Conservationists." United Plant Savers. March 2017. unitedplantsavers.org/the-original -medicinal-plant-gatherers-conservationists.

Axelson, Gustave. "Native Harvest: Ojibwe Wild Rice Gathering in Minnesota." *Midwest Living*. August 17, 2012. midwestliving.com/food/fruits-veggies/native -harvest-ojibwe-wild-rice-gathering-minnesota.

Boughman Arvis Locklear, and Loretta O. Oxendine. *Herbal Remedies of the Lumbee Indians*. Jefferson, NC: McFarland, 2004.

Davenport, Kristen. "Navajo Wild Plants." *Mother Earth Gardener*. August 15, 2021. motherearthgardener.com/profiles/navajo-wild-plant-zmaz15wzsbak.

Deloria, Vine Jr. *God Is Red, A Native View of Religion*. 3rd ed. Golden, CO: Fulcrum Publishing, 2003.

Geniusz, Makoons Wendy. *Our Knowledge Is Not Primitive: Decolonizing Botanical Anishinaabe Teachings*. Syracuse, NY: Syracuse University Press, 2009.

Lapier, Rosalyn R. "Why Is Water Sacred to Native Americans?" *Open Rivers* 8 (Fall 2017): 122–126. openrivers.lib.umn.edu/article/why-is-water-sacred-to -native-americans.

Moerman, Daniel A. *Native American Medicinal Plants, An Ethnobotanical Dictionary: Medicinal Uses of More Than 3,000 Plants by 218 Native American Tribes*. Portland, OR: Timber Press, 2009.

Salmon, Enrique. *Iwigara: American Indian Ethnobotanical Traditions and Science*. Timber Press, 2020.

Shimer, Porter. *Healing Secrets of the Native Americans*. New York: Black Dog & Leventhal, 2004.

Sutherland, A. "Cedar—Sacred Tree with Medicine Power in Native American Beliefs." Ancient Pages. January 6, 2018. ancientpages.com/2018/01/06/cedar -sacred-tree-medicine-power-native-american-beliefs.

Tenny, Louise M. H. *Today's Herbal Health: The Essential Reference Guide*. 6th ed. Salt Lake City, UT: Woodland Publishing, 2007.

Wallace, Eric J. "The Indigenous Tribes Fighting to Reclaim Stevia from Coca-Cola." Atlas Obscura. July 12, 2019. atlasobscura.com/articles/where-is-stevia-from.

Zolbrod, Paul G. *Diné Bahane': The Navajo Creation Story*. Albuquerque, NM: University of New Mexico Press, 1987.

INDEX

A

Abdominal pain
  Diarrhea-Relief Tea, 62
Abenaki, 54
Aches and pains
  Fresh Wild Lettuce Tincture, 66
  Goldthread and Turmeric Electuary, 63
  Herbal-Infused Oil for Pain, 64
  Jamaican Dogwood Tea, 65
Adaptogens, 129
Air element, 10
Alfalfa, 123
Algonquin, 49, 51, 87
Allergy Tea with Goldenrod, 67
Alteratives, 87, 111
American Herbalists Guild, 13
American Indian Religious Freedom Act, 5
Angelica Elixir, 102–103
Anise hyssop, 30, 70
Anishinaabe, 48
Anthocyanins, 80
Antibacterial Healing Herb Liniment, 131
Anxiety
  Passionflower Stress-Relief Tea, 68
  Skullcap Nerve-Support Tea, 69
  Tension-Release Tea, 70
Apache, 52
Astragalus, 106
Aztecs, 51

B

Baby Balm, 132–133
Bacopa, 74
Bark, harvesting tips for, 22
Bartram, William, 57
Baskets, gathering, 20
Beets, 91

Blackberry, 62
Black cohosh, 31, 119
Black Cohosh Tea, 119
Blackfoot, 10, 39
Black haw, 32, 121
Black Haw and Cramp Bark Relief Decoction, 121
Blood pressure
  Heart-Strength Tea, 71
Blood-sugar support
  Homemade Stevia Extract, 72
Blue vervain, 101
Bone broths, 124–125
Bone Health Super Infusion, 123
Boneset, 33, 75
Boneset Tea, 75
Brushes, foraging, 19
Burdock, 7, 34, 86, 91, 134
Burdock and Rosemary Skin and Hair Rinse, 134

C

Cahuilla, 86
Calendula, 108, 132
California poppy, 35, 113
Cardinal directions, 6
Carminatives, 102
Cartier, Jacques, 42
Catnip, 36, 97
Catnip Glycerite, 97
Cattail, 37, 90
Cedar, 7, 8, 56
Chaga fungi, 38, 105
Chaga-Infused Instant Latte, 105
Chamomile, 7, 62, 100, 101
Champlain, Samuel de, 49
Chaparral, 86
Cherokee, 33, 34, 36, 42, 44, 54, 55, 69,
    71, 85, 87, 92, 95, 109, 113, 130, 135

Cheyenne, 30, 39, 49, 138

Children, dosage calculation for, 13

Chinook, 49

Chippewa, 34, 50, 55

Chokecherry, 39, 79

Cholesterol
 Hawthorn-Ginkgo Extract, 73

Cinnamon, 65

Coast Salish, 7

Cognitive function
 Memory Support Tea, 74

Cold and flu
 Boneset Tea, 75
 Elderflower Lemonade, 76
 Pine Tip Tea, 78
 Spiced Chokecherry Syrup, 79
 Triple Lemon Tea, 77
 Wild Violet Sugar, 81
 Winterberry Tea, 80

Constipation-Relief Pastilles, 82

Corn, 40

Corn silk, 104

Cotton root, 41, 120

Cotton-Root Bark Tincture, 120

Cough
 Ground Ivy Respiratory Syrup, 83
 Honeysuckle Cough Syrup, 84
 Wild Ramp Cough Syrup, 85

Cowlitz, 34

Cramp bark, 121

Creek, 57

Cree, 30, 38, 142

D

Dakota, 42

Dandelion, 86, 87, 143

Dandelion Bitters Tincture, 87

Decoctions, 12, 119

Delaware, 34, 36, 69

Denesuliné, 38

Detox
 Potent Detox Tea with Chaparral, 86

Diarrhea-Relief Tea, 62

Digestion
 Dandelion Bitters Tincture, 87
 Fireweed Simple Syrup, 88–89
 Quick Pickled Cattails, 90
 Roasted Burdock Root and Beets, 91

Dosage calculation, 13, 15

Drying methods, 24–25

Duke, James A., 32

E

Ear health
 Mullein Flower Ear Oil, 92

Earth element, 10

Eastern red cedar, 42

Echinacea, 43, 108

Elderberries, 80, 106

Elderberry Syrup, 106

Elderberry tree, 44

Elderflower Lemonade, 76

Electuaries, 63, 118

Elements, 9–11

Eleuthero, 129

Endangered species, 18

Energy
 Healthy Energy Herbal Balls, 93
 Strengthening Iron Tonic, 94
 Yaupon Tea or "Black Drink," 95

Environment
 Milkweed Seed Bombs, 96

F

"The Farm Effect" study, 19

Fenugreek, 115

Fire element, 10

Fireweed, 45, 88

Fireweed Simple Syrup, 88–89

First aid
 Goldenrod Salve, 98–99

Flathead, 52, 82

Foraging. See Wildcrafting

Fresh Wild Lettuce Tincture, 66

Fruits, harvesting tips for, 22

G

Galactologues, 115

Gardening, 14, 24, 25

Garlic, 92

Gas and bloating
  Catnip Glycerite, 97
  Gas-Relief Tea, 100

Gas-Relief Tea, 100

Geniusz, Wendy Makoona, 36, 47, 81

Ginger, 62, 84, 86, 119

Ginkgo biloba, 73

Ginseng, 116

Glycerites, 97

Goat's rue, 115

Goldenrod, 46, 67, 98

Goldenrod Salve, 98–99

Goldenseal, 18, 131

Goldthread, 63

Goldthread and Turmeric Electuary, 63

Goldthread root, 47

Gotu kola, 74, 122

Gotu Kola Tissue-Regeneration Tea, 122

The Green Pharmacy (Duke), 32

Ground Ivy Respiratory Syrup, 83

Guarana, 93

Guarani people, 72

H

Hair health
  Burdock and Rosemary Skin and
    Hair Rinse, 134

Harvesting. See Wildcrafting

Haudenosaunee, 30, 34, 36, 50, 87, 135

Hawthorn, 71, 73

Hawthorn-Ginkgo Extract, 73

Headaches and migraines
  Stress-Induced Headache Tincture, 101

Healers and healing ceremonies, 5, 9

Healthy Energy Herbal Balls, 93

Heart-Strength Tea, 71

Hemple, C. J., 33

Herbal-Infused Oil for Pain, 64

Herbalism, 4–6, 15, 61

Herbal medicine, benefits of, 6–7, 15

Herb-Infused Bone Broth, 124–125

Hibiscus, 71

History of North Carolina (Lawson), 4

Hoh, 36

Homemade Stevia Extract, 72

Honeysuckle Cough Syrup, 84

Hops, 113

Hormone health
  Angelica Elixir, 102–103
  Saw Palmetto Tincture, 104

Horsemint, 48

Horsetail, 123, 134

Huckleberry, 49, 107

Huckleberry-Basil Shrub, 107

I

Immunity
  Chaga-Infused Instant Latte, 105
  Elderberry Syrup, 106
  Huckleberry-Basil Shrub, 107
  Lymph-Mover Tea, 108
  Prickly Pear Salad Dressing, 110
  Red Clover Tea, 111
  Strawberry and Hibiscus Shrub, 109

Insomnia
  Lady's Slipper Root Decoction, 112
  Serenity Cider, 113
  Sleepy-Time Tincture, 114

In-the-Mood Electuary, 118

Isleta, 86

J

Jamaican Dogwood Tea, 65

Jewelweed Salve, 135

K

Keewaydinoquay, 48

Kiowa, 138

Knives, foraging, 20

L

Lactation-Support Tea, 115

Lady's Slipper Root Decoction, 112

Lakota, 6, 52, 54, 130

Lavender, 68

Lawson, John, 4

Lemon balm, 70, 77, 100, 101

Lemongrass, 77

Lemons, 76

Lemon verbena, 77

Libido

   Lovers' Cacao Liqueur, 116–117

   In-the-Mood Electuary, 118

Licorice Root Throat Spray, 141

Linden, 71

Liniments, 131

Loftis, Michelle, 34

Lousewort, 50, 70

Lovers' Cacao Liqueur, 116–117

Lumbee, 36

Lymph-Mover Tea, 108

M

Maca, 118

Manganese, 123

Materica Medica, 13

Medicinal herbs

   benefits of, 6–7, 15

   dosage calculation, 13, 15

   drying, 24–25

   identifying, 18

   preparations, 11–13

   sourcing rare, 23

   storing, 25

Medicine healers, 5

Medicine wheel, 6, 15

Memory Support Tea, 74

Menominee, 33, 34, 50, 116

Menstrual issues

   Black Cohosh Tea, 119

   Black Haw and Cramp Bark Relief Decoction, 121

   Cotton-Root Bark Tincture, 120

Mesquaki, 33

Micmac, 34

Milkweed Seed Bombs, 96

Miwok, 69

Modern-Day Pemmican, 126

Moerman, Daniel, 96

Mohegan, 44

Motherwort, 71

Mountain Mint Mouthwash, 130

Mullein, 84, 92

Mullein Flower Ear Oil, 92

Muscle/tissue

   Gotu Kola Tissue-Regeneration Tea, 122

N

Native American Medicinal Plants
   (Moerman), 96

Native Americans

   healers and healing ceremonies, 5, 9

   herbalism for, 4–6, 15

   herbal knowledge of, 4

The Natural Pregnancy Book (Romm), 41

Navajo, 7, 43, 53, 138

Nervines, 70

Nez Percé, 49

Nootropics, 74

Nutrition

   Bone Health Super Infusion, 123

   Herb-Infused Bone Broth, 124–125

   Modern-Day Pemmican, 126

   Pineapple Weed and Coconut Granola, 127

   Sumac Lemonade, 128

   Ultimate Tonic Tea, 129

O

Oat straw, 70, 115

Oils, 12

Ojibwe, 36, 38, 42, 69, 116, 140

Omaha, 42

Oral health

   Mountain Mint Mouthwash, 130

Our Knowledge Is Not Primitive (Geniusz), 36

P

Paiute, 58, 86
Parsley, 130
Passionflower, 51, 68
Passionflower Stress-Relief Tea, 68
Pastilles, 82
Pawnee, 42, 52
Pemmican, 126
Pennyroyal Pest Spray, 137
Peppermint, 62, 68, 100, 143
Phytosterols, 118
Pima, 52
Pineapple Weed and Coconut Granola, 127
Pine Tip Tea, 78
Pine trees, 78
Pipsissewa, 142
Plantain Salve, 136
Plants, harvesting tips for, 21–22
Plants Have So Much to Give Us, All We have to Do Is Ask (Geniusz), 81
Ponca, 42
Potawatomi, 7
Potent Detox Tea with Chaparral, 86
Poultices, 12
Prickly pear, 52, 110
Prickly Pear Salad Dressing, 110
Pruners, foraging, 20

Q

Quick Pickled Cattails, 90

R

Ramps, 85
Rappahannock, 42
Red clover, 111, 123
Red Clover Tea, 111
Red raspberry leaf, 7, 115
Respect for the earth, 14
Revitalization, 9
Roasted Burdock Root and Beets, 91
Romm, Aviva, 41
Roots, harvesting tips for, 22

Rose hips, 80, 122
Rosemary, 74, 134

S

Sacred medicines, 7–9
Sage, 7, 8
Sagebrush, 53
Saint-John's-wort, 64
Salish, 45, 56
Salves, 12, 98
Sarsaparilla root, 118
Sateré-Mawé, 93
Saw Palmetto Tincture, 104
Scissors, foraging, 20
Seeds, harvesting tips for, 22
Seminole, 57
Serenity Cider, 113
Shamanism, 5
Shatavari, 118
Shoshone, 52, 58, 86
Shrubs, 107
Simple syrups, 88
Skagit, 34
Skin health
    Antibacterial Healing Herb Liniment, 131
    Baby Balm, 132–133
    Burdock and Rosemary Skin and Hair Rinse, 134
    Jewelweed Salve, 135
    Pennyroyal Pest Spray, 137
    Plantain Salve, 136
    Wild Ramp Cough Syrup, 140
    Yucca Root Liquid Soap, 138–139
Skullcap Nerve-Support Tea, 69
Sleepy-Time Tincture, 114
Slippery elm, 82
Smudging, 9
Sore throat
    Licorice Root Throat Spray, 141
Spearmint, 122, 123
Spiced Chokecherry Syrup, 79
Spirulina, 93
Stevia, 72

Stinging nettle, 7, 54
Storing herbs, best practices for, 25
Storytelling, 10
Strawberry and Hibiscus Shrub, 109
Strengthening Iron Tonic, 94
Stress-Induced Headache Tincture, 101
Sumac, 55, 128
Sumac Lemonade, 128
Sweat ceremonies, 9
Sweat-lodge ceremony, 9
Sweetgrass, 7, 8
Swinomish, 82

T

Taino, 65
Teas, 11–12
Tension-Release Tea, 70
Terpenes, 113
Thoreau, Henry David, 49
Timucua, 95
Tinctures, 12
Titration method of dosage calculation, 13
Tobacco, 7, 8
Travels of William Bartram (Bartram), 57
Treasury of American Indian Herbs, A, 39
Triple Lemon Tea, 77
Tulsi, 74
Turmeric, 63, 122
Tuscarora, 40

U

Ultimate Tonic Tea, 129
United Plant Savers, 18

Urinary support
  Urinary Tract Support Tea, 142
  Water-Release Tea, 143
Uva ursi, 142

V

Valerian, 114
Vinegar infusions, 107

W

Water element, 10
Water-Release Tea, 143
Western cedar tree, 56
White sage, 18
Wildcrafting
  about, 18–19, 25
  respectful, 23, 25
  site selection, 20
  tips, 21–22
  tools, 19–20
Wild lettuce, 66
Wild Ramp Cough Syrup, 85
Wild Rice Skin Exfoliator, 140
Wild Violet Sugar, 81
Winterberry Tea, 80

Y

Yaupon holly, 57, 95
Yaupon Tea or "Black Drink," 95
Yerba santa, 58
Yucca Root Liquid Soap, 138–139
Yurok, 82

Acknowledgments

I would like to thank my teachers Graham Wesley and Rose Fairly from Dwelling Earth Medicine School, both for creating safe spaces to learn. Kat Lee for encouraging me to focus on moving the needle forward for BIPOC writers, and the Lumbee author Arvis Boughman for encouraging me to share our Indigenous plant knowledge.

About the Author

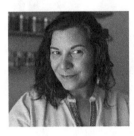 **Angela Locklear Queen** is an enrolled member of the Lumbee Tribe of North Carolina. She has been a student and practitioner of nutrition and herbalism, receiving her certification as a Nutritional Therapy Practitioner and studying herbalism through The Science and Art of Herbalism, Dwelling School of Earth Medicine as well as through Indigenous mentorship.

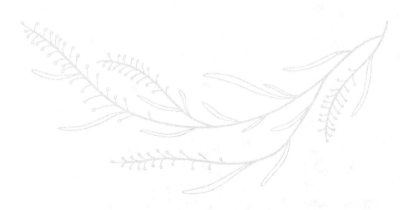

Printed in the USA
CPSIA information can be obtained
at www.ICGtesting.com
CBHW081416270424
7400CB00001B/1

9 798886 501278